COLUMBIA COLLEGE
616.89A456P   C1   V0

PORTRAIT OF THE ARTIST AS A YOUNG PAT

3 2711 00003 7438

616.89 A456p

Alper, Gerald.

Portrait of the arti
young patient

D1767104

ENTERED JUL 1 3 1992

Portrait of the Artist as a Young Patient
Psychodynamic Studies of the Creative Personality

Portrait of the Artist as a Young Patient
Psychodynamic Studies of the Creative Personality

Gerald Alper, M.S.

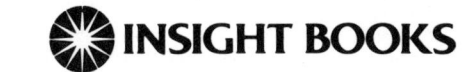
INSIGHT BOOKS

Plenum Press • New York and London

Library of Congress Cataloging-in-Publication Data

```
Alper, Gerald.
    Portrait of the artist as a young patient : psychodynamic studies
  of the creative personality / Gerald Alper.
        p.    cm.
    Includes bibliographical references and index.
    ISBN 0-306-44126-8
    1. Artists--Mental health.  2. Artists--Psychology.
  3. Narcissism.  4. Creative ability.   I. Title.
     [DNLM: 1. Creativeness.  2. Narcissism.  3. Personality.
  4. Psychoanalytic Therapy.    WM 460.5.E3 A456p]
  RC451.4.A7A46  1992
  616.89'008'87--dc20                                   91-35425
                                                            CIP
```

616.89 A456p

Alper, Gerald.

Portrait of the artist as a
young patient

ISBN 0-306-44126-8

©1992 Plenum Press, New York
A Division of Plenum Publishing Corporation
233 Spring Street, New York, N.Y. 10013

An Insight Book

All rights reserved

No part of this book may be reproduced, stored in a retrieval system, or transmitted in any form or by any means, electronic, mechanical, photocopying, microfilming, recording, or otherwise, without written permission from the Publisher

Printed in the United States of America

To my parents
Robert and Gloria

my children
Steve and Tom

and

Anita

Preface

The artist who appears here belongs to a special population of struggling, noncommercial, artist-patients rarely seen in the private office of a psychoanalytic psychotherapist (as is the case here) for the compelling reason that they cannot afford a normal fee. What made these artist-patients accessible to me over the past ten years was an affiliation with an unusual nonprofit organization, Community Guidance Service, which provided both the required sliding scale fee system and the equally important referral source to outside psychotherapists (such as myself) who were willing to abide by it. What follows is not intended as a scholarly review of the many theories of artistic creativity or as a catalogue of treatment issues with artist-patients. In its place, is a presentation of certain salient characteristics that have emerged during my ten years of working with artists who became patients—specifically, a kind of narcissism that manifested itself in a series of unique, narcissistic relationships: the relationship of the artist to his creativity or talent; the relationship of the artist to his teacher; the relationship of the artist to his imagined public; and the relationship of the artist to his therapist.

Over the past ten years, I worked with about thirty artists in individual psychoanalytic psychotherapy, as intensively as I could—allowing for the fact that many artists are highly resistant to therapy. During the same period, I also performed diagnostic intakes for Community Guidance Service, managing to see, on a single-session basis, approximately one hundred additional future artist-patients.

Here is a common, recurring profile of the artist as patient: someone in the mid- to late twenties; more likely female than male but, surprisingly, with a significantly higher percentage of males in comparison to nonartistic patient populations; generally not indigenous to New York City, but arriving and settling in from the Tristate area, from the Midwest, and even from California; either being or aspiring to be an actor, actress, musician, dancer, painter, singer, or writer; generally unemployed in his craft and having to fall back on part-time survival work such as waiting tables in restaurants (almost unanimously despised); predominant presenting problem of depression (often narcissistic), work inhibition, creative block, paralysis of initiative, "will power," and day-to-day functioning, accompanied by frequent feelings of inner deadness.

The patients whose stories are described here come from a variety of socioeconomic backgrounds, but they were united in that they were all poor (unable to sustain themselves in their chosen professions), and all felt defeated by the overwhelming competitiveness of the subculture that is the artistic life-style in New York City. This creative, artistic personality, although usually portrayed in the literature as superficially successful, is a favorite type of narcissistic personality often cited by prominent writers on the subject of pathological narcissism (Kernberg 1975, 1986; Kohut 1971; Miller 1981) but typically accorded no special treatment, merely being mentioned as one of a series of types.

A somewhat different view will be presented in this book: that the narcissism of the artist is unique in that it receives a kind of special intensity of reinforcement (both intrapsychic and interpersonal) that generally does not occur in other narcissistic personalities. The artistic narcissism to be delineated is *not* intended as a clinical, differential diagnosis: although all of the patients described herein were, to some extent, narcissistic personalities, each of them also manifested clearcut borderline symptoms, and none of them fit comfortably into either a familiar Kohut (1971) or Kernberg (1975) categorization of narcissistic or borderline pathology. Instead, it is suggested that the artist is a highly *atypical* patient, and his narcissism (neither healthy nor pathological, but a mixture of both), rather than being an explanatory model for the etiology of creativity, or even a neurotic by-product of it, is, instead—as will be shown—a necessary, intrinsic part of the artistic process itself.

Acknowledgments

First, I would like to thank the anonymous reader at the *Psychoanalytic Review* who was assigned my initial entry into the field, and who delighted me by wholeheartedly endorsing it. Encouraged, I wrote another, then another, gradually making a transition, after a lapse of years, from a writer of short stories, someone who wrote fiction about people, to someone who wrote about people unhappily enmeshed in their own psychical fictions.

Although I have had my share of inspirational teachers, I have learned the most by far from my patients, typified by the patient who one afternoon—after my searching for years to find my own voice as a therapist—jarred me by noting, "You've changed," and went on to explain that somehow I seemed more accessible to her and more at ease with myself.

From an entirely different, and much more personal perspective, I drew inspiration from the fact that both my sons are starting out on the track of being young artists and that by devoting a book to the struggles of young artists, I was also, perhaps in a vicarious father-and-sons way, participating in their adventure.

Every writer needs a receptive audience of at least one, hopefully someone other than himself. Anita was my audience. She was with me from the very first paper I wrote for the *Psychoanalytic Review*, the first proposal I wrote for this book, the first chapter up until the very last, and is still with me. Her enthusiastic, nurturing belief in the worth of what I was doing, even during times when I myself was uncertain, was a vital stimulant to continue.

I would like to thank my editor, Norma Fox, who, amidst a sea of proposals which I imagine regularly inundates publishers, managed to find me. Her strong, unambivalent support was both a relief and comfort, allowing me to plunge ahead with the projected work much more confidently than I had ever imagined.

And I must not forget Sandra Davis-Randle, my friend, who, fortunately for me, is not only an expert word processor but also a conscientious one. At times, she amazed me by being even more faithful to the accuracy and integrity of the printed word than I was.

Contents

Chapter 1
The Artist Comes to Therapy   1

Steve, the Magical Pianist   3
The Relationship of the Artist to His Talent and
    to His Audience   12
The Artist in Psychotherapy   16
The Double Bind of the Artist in Psychotherapy   17

Chapter 2
Yesterday's Narcissism   29

Early Hopes   31
The Dream Fades   33
The Last Session   36
The Will to Survive   41

Chapter 3
Creative Paranoia 45

The Third Degree 47
Dan, the Would-Be Rock Star 57
A Bad Trip with The Grateful Dead 65
The Paranoid Companion 86
Intimacy Panic 89

Chapter 4
The Death of an Artist 99

Harry's Denial 101
When You Know You're About to Die 115
The Good Soldier 117
The Impact of Certain Death on the Psyche 122

Chapter 5
The Painterly Eye 137

Marie's Two Worlds 139
The Bridge 142
The Schizoid Artist 146
The Disappointing Real World 154

Chapter 6
If Wittgenstein Were a Patient 157

The Tortured Young Philosopher 159
The Mystery of the Unsaid 163
Escaping from the Paranoid Style 167
Wittgenstein and Psychoanalysis 169

Chapter 7
The Psychoanalyst: As True and False Self   *177*

As a Candidate   *180*
As a Faculty Supervisor   *181*
As a Famous Analyst   *183*
The Flight from Unreality   *189*
The Good Enough Analyst   *197*

Chapter 8
The Double Bind in Psychoanalysis   *199*

The Analyst's Dilemma   *204*
An Artificial Human Laboratory   *206*
The First Therapeutic Double Standard   *209*
Transference and the Double Bind   *212*

Conclusion   *215*

Making It   *217*
The Young Artist as Prototype   *219*

Glossary   *221*

References   *229*

Index   *235*

1
The Artist Comes to Therapy

STEVE, THE MAGICAL PIANIST

A clinical vignette which made a vivid impression on me can perhaps best illustrate what I consider special about the narcissism of the artist. This particular artist had been a patient of mine for about three years, and throughout all of that time he had been painfully shy, self-doubting, self-tormenting, and always managing to suffer intensely in just about every facet of his life. There was only one thing Steve felt he was good at: the piano. As part of a family of musical overachievers, he had found himself entered in local piano competitions from the age of eight onward and it was a rare occasion when he didn't win. By the time he was twenty, he was entering and doing outstandingly well in international piano competitions. By the time Steve entered therapy with me, at the age of twenty-three, he had already been identified by his musical peers (in print) as a leading young American pianist. That was the good news. The bad news was that Steve could barely live; did not know how to take care of himself; subsisted on handouts from his parents and part-time work as a waiter, and found himself unable to initiate even the first step toward the chosen career for which he seemed almost predestined—that of concert pianist. Instead, Steve elected to use therapy as a vehicle to shore up what he considered a deplorable lack of "assertiveness" in himself. Indeed, after several years of therapeutic work a high point for Steve came when, uncharacteristically, he refused to accommodate the request of a customer at a catered party who had asked him to fold up a tablecloth, condescendingly alluding to Steve as a "professional tablecloth folder." "No," replied Steve, curtly, as he proudly walked away, "I am *not* a professional tablecloth folder."

The incident, which produced such a vivid impression on me, occurred a few months prior to the termination of therapy. Unexpectedly, in the midst of a session, Steve offered me complimentary tickets to a concert hall in New York City where he was scheduled to make his debut as a solo pianist. Although I had been trained, analytically, to generally avoid such extratherapeutic activities as unwanted parameters to the treatment, I did not hesitate to accept: feeling, first, that to turn down the invitation would do more harm than good to the therapy (in the way of unexplainable narcissistic injury), and, second, being secretly pleased as I could not help but be curious and eager to witness the performing persona I had heard so much about.

Accordingly, several days later I found myself packed into an audience of several hundred people, all anticipating the entrance of my patient. As I began to share in the gathering excitement, I also began, involuntarily, to recollect memories of our sessions. For three years, Steve had steadily radiated almost complete psychic helplessness and inadequacy. Intellectually, I knew he was a fine pianist whom this sophisticated-looking audience was likely to appreciate. But how, I wondered, would he ever muster that inner command and psychic presence needed to *move* them emotionally? The more I empathized with the secret inner life of the patient I imagined I thoroughly knew, the uneasier I became.

The Artist Comes to Therapy

Steve's entrance, when it came, only accelerated my anxiety. He appeared in a suit I knew was a hand-me-down from an older brother that was still one or two sizes too big for him. He walked sheepishly across the bare stage. Seating himself at the piano, Steve suddenly—with his familiar self-torturing indecisiveness—began to wonder if the height of his stool was correct. For about two minutes, as the audience waited, Steve repeatedly raised the stool, then lowered it—obviously unable to make up his mind. The uneasiness that I felt was now spreading to the audience. In the subsequent session, Steve would confide to me that he only stopped obsessing about the proper height of his stool when he sensed the audience was on the brink of erupting into "nervous giggling." So at that precise moment, Steve stopped, composed himself, and decided it was time to play. Except it was more like exploding, as he would later put it, "into my musical space." In what seemed an instant, Steve had not only crashed the opening, thunderous chord but had traversed the length of the keyboard with astonishing speed. Immediately captured, the audience grew still. For the next twenty minutes, through thousands of notes, slightly leaning forward in a kind of vigilant, trancelike state, my patient delivered a dazzling exhibition of performing virtuosity. At its conclusion, two elderly women sitting immediately in front of me—apparent habitués of recital halls—jointly shook their heads: "That was incredible, just incredible," whispered one of them. What was more incredible to me than the obvious technical expertise was the fact that for twenty minutes I had been witnessing someone I scarcely knew; someone who, seemingly, in a magical moment had metamorphosed from a person of great psychic fragility into a being of stately, almost godlike self-assurance.

Leaving the concert hall, I could only wonder what it was that had effected such a psychic metamorphosis. The conventional answer that it was attributable to his "genius" or his "talent" only seemed to beg the question. To a certain extent what follows is, in part, my attempt at an answer.

Although not all my artist-patients possessed the talent of a Steve, and there was the expected range of variation, the characteristic that most singled them out as a group was their creative talent. Whether innate or acquired, their creativity was appreciable and clearly above the norm. If we compare the creative talent of an artist with that of the ordinary nonartistic person (as I often had the opportunity to do within my own practice)—and measure it in the light of the special talents and healthy narcissism (Kohut 1977) which every person has in some measure—certain immediate differences arise. Artistic talent, compared to the average, is a much more powerful, readily available, immediate narcissistic supply and, as in the case of Steve, a sometimes magical-seeming force which, in its ability to enhance and energize, can narcissistically empower an otherwise fluctuating self-esteem. In this sense, artistic talent is *transformative*; and because it is so effectively transformative it can even serve as a psychic substitute for some of the self-regulating soothing functions associated (especially in dependent people) with the infusion of external drugs (Krystal 1973). Yet, from the viewpoint we are presenting, the creativity of the artist is more potent than a powerful drug, being that it is even more readily available inasmuch as it is an internal function, subject to psychic control—that can be psychically produced—rather than the other way around; which means that creativity can be passive in its relationship to the psyche instead of the psyche being passive to the effects of foreign drugs. If we take our comparison of talent and drugs one step further and apply it to the concept of healthy narcissism (Kohut 1977), we see some immediate advantages: the exercise of artistic talent—far from implying toxic side effect, hangover, psychic debilitation, depressed crashing—may even contribute to the building of psychic structure. We also see some negative, analogous effects: for example, the trancelike rapture of being engaged in flowing creative work can feel like being "stoned," while the postpartum depression that sometimes follows a sustained creative effort may experientially get confused with drug-related "crashing." What is more, if we compare talent from the perspective of familiar, fast-acting drugs, there are clear-cut disadvantages: instead of guaranteed highs and quick relief, there is long hard work, delayed gratification, and painstaking reality testing. There are highs in the production of legitimate art, but (as most artists will tell you) they are few and far between; so, it is not surprising that many artists (as was true with most of my patients), perhaps to compensate for this, use (and often abuse) drugs as a kind of auxiliary narcissistic backup, that is, for those times when talent fails.

The relationship of the artist to his talent can be confused, complex, and ambivalent. An artist may have particular trouble delimiting the boundaries of his talent. An artist may feel his talent to be so overflowing that he is unclear as to whether his talent is in him, or whether, in terms of Bion's container (1975), he is somehow in his talent: driven, possessed, contained by it. So compelling, so likely to overflow and take him over, it may seem to the artist that his regular self were somehow subordinate to a higher, supraordinated artistic self: experientially something like Kohut's supraordinated self (1977, p. 97). Seen in this light, the reverse of this, work inhibition or creative blocking, is not hard to understand. When talent shrinks to something small and impotent, as though the psychic battery which powers the self has gone dead, it can mean to artists the effective strangulation of their chief narcissistic source of animating energy. They often experience it as a profound cancellation of their basic life force. Therefore, when your patient is an artist, it can be particularly difficult to determine whether, as is sometimes the case, a depression has preceded the work inhibition and creative blocking—or has followed it. In other words, creative blocking can be so psychically debilitating to an artist that a serious depression can be an almost appropriate reactive depression. Finally, because so much of self and identity is concentrated in the artistic self, creative blocking can be experienced as almost a *suicide of the self*. In a real sense, creatively blocked artists, artists who have outlived their talent, often feel useless and without self-justifying worth in a way reminiscent of patients suffering from true survivor's guilt.

It follows that a relationship as important, powerful, and intense as that which exists between the artist and his talent must find representation in the transference. It does. Transferentially, artists tend not to be as interested in insight as they are in stimulation and gratification. The insight they seem to treasure most is of the "Ah-hah!" kind, with a minimum of follow-up cognitive processing and working through. In therapy, they tend to be restless, bored, and, in varying degrees, generally detached. Their presence is distinctly not what one stereotype would have it: charismatic. Of course, this may be partially due to the fact that they are bringing their sick self and not their performing, creative self to therapy. Positive and negative transferences often revolve around the degree of narcissistic supply projectively identified with in their therapist. For example, patients who perceived my low-key and thoughtful style (at least as I believe it is) as basically undynamic and unenergetic formed negative transferences to me.

Tom, an intellectualizing, withdrawn, and rather hopeless young musician, periodically confided to me that while he appreciated that I was "very intelligent and comfortable to talk to," what he probably really needed in order to get well was a group like EST to rehaul his psyche.

Elizabeth, a beautiful, agitated, hysterically impulsive actress who managed to fail at whatever job she landed, who experienced her considerable talent as almost chaotic, demonic, and alien, told me that while "I was a nice man whom she had absolutely nothing against," the one who could turn everything around and redeem her suffering was Norman Vincent Peale (whom she tried in vain to see).

Christopher, a very belligerent young actor-playwright who was openly contemptuous of anything he felt blocked his way, once flatly appraised me (referring to what he perceived as my almost zero charisma): "You? *You're dead!*"

In the transference (whether positive or negative) talent can be used as resistance. Often artists try to isolate, separate, and protect their talent from the treatment. On the one hand, they want their therapists to admire and appreciate their creative work; on the other hand, they do not necessarily want them to come close to it, inspect it (as audience), for fear of contamination. The relationship is intensely ambivalent: they want to disguise and camouflage their talent and also, when the timing is right, to dramatically unveil it. Sometimes, artists want their therapists to almost symbiotically know that they are gifted without needing to demonstrate it. They then secretly study their therapist for clues which can indicate if they are truly aware of the depth of their patient's talent, using it as a test of trust on the part of their therapist: that is, if my therapist really understands, likes, and trusts me, he *knows* I am a fine artist.

Creativity is such an integral part of an artist's identity that it is almost impossible to believe that an important person like their therapist can dislike their art (whether on aesthetic or personal grounds) and not also dislike them. Conversely, when artists need distance from their therapist, it may take the form of a defensive need to believe that the therapist could not possibly understand or like their art. Should these patients come to believe that their therapist finally does understand both them and their art, it can then represent a terrifying excess of closeness and a threat of engulfment. Such a patient was Marie, a tall, proud woman of vibrant intelligence and an artist-designer of exquisite taste. Although devoted for four years to her therapy and to me, on more than one occasion she would roll her eyes around my office and coolly pronounce, "This must be one of the ugliest rooms in the world." When at last she felt, sadly, it was time to leave therapy and go off on her own she revealed to me, as gently as she could, that there was an intractable chasm between us created by her artistic sensibility, and therefore things she knew she could never even begin to try to explain to me. As close as I felt to and as well as I thought I knew Marie, I realized to my surprise that she had a genuine need (which she rather enjoyed satisfying) to see me as a bit of a philistine.

Time and again I was struck by how fiercely and possessively artists tried to isolate and protect their talent in therapy. One way to understand this is to think of the concept of ego splitting (Freud 1938; Kernberg 1975) and apply it to the idea of the artist's special sense of an artistic self. We then get the brief formula of bad art = bad self and good art = good self. Another way of saying this is that the development of the artistic identity will tend to lag *behind* (that is, be more primitive) than the development of the remainder of the psyche. In this regard, we are reminded of Erik Erikson's telling observation (1959) that the creative identity of artists is unusual in that, in a certain sense, it is perpetually unfinished. Most of my clinical experience with artists validated this: predominantly, their identity issues tended to be the ones that were especially unresolved. Sometimes, when the discrepancy and tension between conflicting levels of identity development—between the artistic and nonartistic self—become too acute, a defensive false self (Winnicott 1960) can arise. This can occur in several ways. When the artistic identity is so hyperdeveloped as to be far ahead of the rest of the personality, as was the case with my pianist, Steve, there may be a false self in the sense that the artist generally feels unworthy of the attention lavished by audiences on his talent. As Steve meekly put it to me, "I'm always surprised to find people in awe of me. After all, what I do on the piano, to me is like brushing my teeth." Alternatively, an artist may be confused as to which is the false self (his artistic self or his nonartistic self); and, if especially artistically insecure, may—through projective identification—collude with the shallow narcissistic appreciation of an overimpressed audience and willingly mistake it for authentic reinforcement of his artistic true self (Winnicott 1960).

Just as there are special transferential issues between artist and therapist, there are corresponding, if not always congruent, countertransferential issues (Raecker 1968). For example, therapists working with artists can experience an inordinate demand for validation, encouragement, and performance. In part, this may be due to the fact that the specialness which every patient searches for, to some degree, in his therapist is magnified in the artist. While they do not necessarily seek out therapists who share their interests—as, for example, other atypical patient populations (recovering alcoholics, gays) often do—and may even prefer nonartistic therapists (so as to avoid painful narcissistic competition), they are usually more insistent than most patients on a feeling of specialness in the therapists they choose. The artist as patient can be easily repelled by what he considers a conventionality and ordinariness of sensibility in his therapist, and often will react to any intervention smacking of textbook technique as though it were a narcissistic injury. The therapist has to steer a delicate course here: to resist pressure from the artist to excessively (and without basis in reality) affirm an unseen talent, and the corresponding countertransferential need to be empathic and supportive in the area most essential to the artist's self-esteem. Reality testing (on the part of the therapist) is more important when your patient is an artist: since so much of an artist's identity and self-esteem is riding on his talent, there is added countertransferential pressure to try to objectively assess it.

This is hard enough to do, when the therapist is only going by the artist's subjective reports. Yet, if there is an invitation or opportunity to personally review the work, a new countertransferential issue immediately crops up. Is it helpful to the artist for the therapist to accept the role of involuntary art critic or enlisted member of the audience? How honest should the therapist be if he really dislikes the art (which would be devastating to the artist)? In ten years of working with artists, I was asked on three occasions (in addition to my pianist) to personally witness the work. In each instance, after some initial indecision, I ventured to trust my sense of the patient (each of whom also knew me well before asking) that I would genuinely be able to find something pleasing in their work. In each case, my intuition was validated. I not only liked their work on a personal, aesthetic basis, but I managed to derive extra satisfaction, an almost parental, nurturing feeling (or fantasy) that I had partially contributed to their achievement. I subsequently realized that since these patients could not have gauged my personal artistic tastes, their requests transferentially revealed a level of trust, a belief that I would at least be a receptive, nurturing audience who would give their work a rooting chance; and they felt good enough about themselves and their creativity in the context of our relationship, to gamble on their art and take their chances with it. Seen in this light, it was no coincidence that all of my artist-patients who specifically went out on the limb and asked me to look at their work, had very positive transferences to me. The corollary of this, of course, is that an artist's continued withdrawal of work or references to work from therapy, can be a serious indication of negative transference (mistrust).

One personal, countertransferential issue: since I had a background as a published novelist and short story writer, I occasionally had the impulse to share this with my artists and to say, in effect, "I, too, am an artist. I know what you're going through because I went through it, too." Yet I always resisted this, my intuition telling me that in the dyad of artist–therapist—especially unemployed, often unrecognized artist—there was room for only one talent to narcissistically shine.

THE RELATIONSHIP OF THE ARTIST TO HIS TALENT AND TO HIS AUDIENCE

Artistic talent, the special powers of creativity possessed by the genuine artistic temperament—in its seeming ability to transcend boundaries, imaginatively rearrange reality, multiply the self by assuming other identities, and perhaps, most of all, shock ordinary people with its finished product into a kind of admiring trance—may experientially be perceived by the artist as a kind of objective omnipotent-feeling grandiose self (Kohut). In "The Relation of the Poet to Daydreaming" (1908), Freud emphasized the poet's ability—by protectively wrapping up infantile, aggressive, sexual, and narcissistic wishes in aesthetic covers—to awaken in ordinary people similar repressed desires. We can only add, how much more evocative is the artist's (poet's) ability to summon forth from his own unconscious these same desires; that is, to either evocatively, associatively intensify or regressively return to early grandiose self-images. We can sum this up by saying that in *psychic reality artistic creativity feels magical and can be equivalent to a grandiose self.*

If this is so, then what of the relationship of the artistic process to its audience? We may understand this better if we recognize that the artistic process must always essentially involve the *externalization of normal self-esteem and its placement in the hands of a critically powerful, unknown, detached public (no matter how select) who function as a deciding jury.* To this degree, there is something opposing the normal development of internalization of self-esteem resulting in healthy narcissism, and is instead conducive to a relationship between artist and public, described by Kohut (1971), as selfobject. Yet there is a remarkable difference. There is another sense, a reality sense, in which the relationship between artist and public resembles *an objective (i.e., healthy, nonpathological) selfobject.* It is objective because many of the traits Kohut attributes to the psychic selfobject (1971) do in fact *objectively* describe aspects of the artist's relationship to his audience. The artist is symbiotic with his audience in the sense that no artist can actualize the creative process without the necessary validation of a critical public; the artist is objectively symbiotic with his audience in the sense that his self-worth cannot come from himself alone, that is, no artist has ever been accorded worth (whether contemporaneously or posthumously) if no one other than the artist thought so; by contrast there are many pathological narcissists who are essentially alone in the high value they place on themselves. Summing up, we can say that *the artist and his audience are like an objective selfobject in that they cannot logically exist apart in the developmental, psychic sense that may be said of self and object in healthy narcissistic development* (Kohut 1977).

Seen in this light, there is an interesting comparison between how Freud spoke of the group (1921) and the relationship of the artist to his public we are trying to depict. According to Freud (1921), the group leader captures the ego-ideal of the individual as does the beloved: in both cases the ego-ideal *moves outside* the individual. Now something like the reverse of this formula is what happens to the artist in relation to his public. *The public captures the ego-ideal of the artist and to that extent assumes the character of a beloved (and must be pursued).*

If this is so, what of the relationship of the audience to artist? The artist–audience relationship is striking in how radically asymmetrical it is. The audience is almost completely receptive. It has no input. It patiently assembles and waits to be stimulated. It is not allowed to respond beyond its anticipated appreciation. It cannot interact and its responses are carefully programmed in advance by the performing artist. Should the audience respond with a negative reception (lack of appreciation)—which may be significant from the standpoint of reality testing—it will generally be considered by the artist as a narcissistic injury and almost never a constructive criticism. Seen in this light, if the artist occupies something like the position of an objective grandiose self in relationship to the audience, then, reciprocally, the audience's narcissism must shrink. To the degree the audience experiences itself in the role of appreciative handmaiden to the artist's grandiose self *it must suffer a continuous narcissistic injury* which it tries *to cover up with escalating demands for narcissistic gratification (to be fed ever more satisfying and grandiose works of art).*

Perhaps nothing shows the relationship of artist to public as clearly as that of the performing artist to live audience (because it is in pure form). The performing artist asks not only to be related to, but to be loved. In the sense that the artist wants to be loved, the type of object choice he aspires to is narcissistic (Freud 1914). The audience understands this, as well as the implication that there is a symbiosis between artist and audience in which—though each has very different roles—both will partake deeply of the performance to come. The performance begins in expectation and almost Messianic high hope (Bion 1974) for the audience. The obvious narcissism of the performer excites them not only in the way the sight of blatant, successful narcissists excite them (Freud 1914). It far surpasses that. From the perspective of the audience, the performing artist—a narcissist who does not simply seek out the love of many, but appears confident of getting it and objectively worthy of receiving it—is a kind of heroic, super grandiose self. The implied symbiosis, the sense that the artist urgently needs the participation and cooperative love of the audience, only heightens the illusion that the audience is about to receive substantial narcissistic supplies. This illusion—no matter how willing the suspension of disbelief, no matter how artistically seductive the performer—has to dwindle. The artist urgently needs but cannot care for, certainly does not know, and even if he had the capacity does not have the time to reciprocally admire the audience. By the nature of the artistic process, the artist has been placed in a kind of double bind, an impossible position: he is to reveal a deep part of himself, to be symbolically intimate with an anonymous crowd. Far from loving and relating to the audience, the artist, once he has used up the narcissistic supply of one audience, must hurry on to the next narcissistic supply. After eliciting the hoped-for appreciative love of his audience, he can no longer offer his public anything. To his audience, he can begin to assume the guise of an *aesthetic Don Juan*. In the sense that the artistic process creates a necessary relationship between artist and public that allows of no other interaction than initial contact and impact between artist and public followed only by (hoped for) appreciative love of a particular audience, *the artist, whether he wants to or not, is doomed to a narcissistic relationship*. Gradually, the audience understands this. The impersonality of the relationship sooner or later becomes apparent and therein somewhat frightening. It dawns on the audience that while it is needed, it is needed as an object (Khan 1979), an implement for the artist's primary need to be artistically gratified. From this perception of narcissistic injury at being used, there is a regression to its own grandiose self: the audience defensively craves more and more narcissistic supplies (feedings of ever more glorious art) and restores itself, soothes its narcissistic injury suffered at the hands of the artist by becoming increasingly, more aggressively demanding.

We can sum this up by saying that *the dynamic of the relationship between artist and public, from the viewpoint we are presenting, is a symbiosis of reciprocal selfobjects: a selfobject that is more objective and rooted in reality on the part of the artist in its relationship to its public; and a selfobject that is more reactive, regressive, and archaic on the part of the public in its relationship to the artist.*

The Artist in Psychotherapy

By the time the artist arrives in therapy, there usually has already occurred (especially in professional artists in New York City) *an early narcissistic defeat*. The loss that the artist has sustained, often beginning in the late twenties, differs from the sense of physiological loss at the onset of middle age with its prospect of inevitable, accelerated aging and decline. Instead, the artist has begun to succumb to the reality and weight of a unique series of greater narcissisms: the narcissism, for example, of the acting teacher who will often manipulate the actor for his own narcissistic gain; the narcissism of the auditioning casting director who can possess almost complete and sometimes dehumanizing control over the fate and (more importantly) dignity of the artist; and, most significantly, the narcissism of the industry itself, so thoroughly and commercially self-absorbed, as to be immune to the delicate emotional needs of the subordinate and powerless artists.

The loss that the artist sustains, then, is a loss of narcissistic hope. The artist begins to realize and try to accommodate to a life where professional employment is likely to be episodic, meager, and less than self-supporting. There is a demoralizing sense that the artist who has staked his self-esteem on his art, who has put all of his eggs, so to speak, in one basket is not only going to come up short but is going to come up empty. This may be why the narcissistic deflation of artists often takes the guise of crashing from a drug-induced high; and why the presenting clinical symptom of many artists is (narcissistic) depression. As a result, the artist entering therapy is more and more estranged from his former narcissism, which now appears ego dystonic to him. More and more, artists find that instead of motivating themselves, they have to psych themselves up, especially for anxiety-producing personal encounters such as auditions, which are increasingly dreaded. A common complaint is to wonder at the loss of their former supply of narcissistic energy, which they express as a loss of confidence. They begin to mourn their lost narcissism.

Now the artist is disillusioned and no longer reinforced in his specialness, and can confront the underlying human problems he has in common with other nonartistic patients. For the first time, therapy can move to a more hopeful and real level.

THE DOUBLE BIND OF THE ARTIST IN PSYCHOTHERAPY

As conceived by Gregory Bateson (Bateson et al. 1956) the double bind was thought to arise from a nexus of paradoxical, mixed messages and conflicting levels of communication. In contrast to this, we view the therapeutic double bind as arising from a conflict of incompatible levels of intimacy: specifically, the (unspoken of) conflict between technique and intimacy (Alper 1991). Seen in this light, the central double bind, from the viewpoint of the therapeutic dyad, is that the patient is put into the role (or expectation) of nonreciprocal intimacy with a professional stranger. The central double bind from the standpoint of the therapist is that, in a dyadic setting often evocative of profound intimacy, he is constrained to behave in a manner largely dictated by an impersonal, professional technique (regardless of how empathically that technique may be delivered).

These two factors—the special narcissism of the artist and the double bind of the therapeutic process—combine to produce a series of unique double binds for the artist who enters psychotherapy.

Long before the artist enters psychotherapy, he is prone to a double bind most of us do not suffer from. The principal double bind of the artist is that he attempts, symbolically, to be intimate (express a deep part of his personality) with an anonymous crowd. Perhaps it is the intrinsic impossibility of such a relationship that creates the need in the artist's personality to sometimes fall back upon (or regress) to narcissism as a compensatory defense.

Too much attention has been paid to the risk and courage it takes to reveal oneself as an artist, and not enough to the fact that once an artist has symbolically expressed himself in the deepest way he can, that is, once he has made contact and initiated a relationship with the audience, his contribution is finished. The artist's relationship to his public so far as *his* input goes, ends immediately after it begins. Once the artist elicits the hoped-for appreciative love of his audience, he can no longer offer his public anything.

The relationship of the artist to his intended public therefore is a peculiar one—a kind of symbolic, elusive intimacy. In a certain Winnicottian sense (1953), the symbolic intimacy of the artist might be looked upon not as a transitional object, but as a transitional level of intimacy (intermediate between playing and reality). The process of artistic creation and expression may serve ambivalent needs: the artist expresses something deep, personal, and creatively spontaneous, yet relates it in a style that is profoundly and formally deliberate. On the one hand, what the artist expresses could not be more intensely personal; on the other hand the object to whom he expresses it (audience) could not be more distant and impersonal. Looked at this way, the relationship of the artist to his creativity is also narcissistic inasmuch as the product of his creativity is intended mainly for the benefit (narcissistic enhancement) of the artist and not for the audience. What the artist presents to the audience is a deep part of himself. What he wants in return is admiration and applause; even more significantly, he doesn't really want *any other part of the audience than its praise* and has no further interest in knowing, relating to, or caring about the audience.

In this way, the relationship of the artist to his audience can be seen as a perversion of intimacy (Khan 1979). The audience is reduced by the artistic process to the status of an indispensable tool subserving the narcissistic needs of the artist; while the particular technique of the artist becomes a narcissistic strategy to coerce the audience into gratification of the artist's need. While these are certainly not the truest needs of art they may, at times, be the defensive *uses* of art. The artist who either exposes himself recklessly to an unseen and potentially critically dangerous public or, as a performer, expresses himself directly to an equally demanding audience, may use *narcissism as a defense*. In other words, in order to deeply reveal himself before an anonymous (and thereby invulnerable, unmovable) audience the artist may find it necessary to rely upon a narcissistic relationship: i.e., one that exclusively focuses on the gratification of his own needs, as a necessary defense against the double bind of trying to be symbolically intimate with a faraway, untouchable crowd.

Summing up, art aspires after the appreciative love of its audience in contrast to science which aims at the understanding and consensual validation of its audience. We can only comment that there seems to be something remarkably (and perhaps necessarily) narcissistic in this basic relationship of the artist to his audience. The way an artist can quickly move on from one audience to the next, once he has used up the unique narcissistic supplies of a particular audience, is reminiscent, as previously mentioned, of an aesthetic Don Juan.

What of the relationship of the audience to the artist? On some level, they must recognize the double bind of the artist: that while yearning for the greatest appreciative love through presentation of his art, the artist can only offer the symbolic gift of his art—an almost completely impersonal relationship. Seen in this light, the oft-noted insatiable, willful, and fickle neediness of the public may be explained, partially, as *an act of retaliation*. Artists, for their part, often feel enslaved by what they perceive as the narcissistic demands of their public, and sense that no matter how well they succeed in satisfying them, there will always be a fresh demand for narcissistic supplies. By the same token, audiences may feel entitled to be blatantly narcissistic—to impulsively cheer or hiss according to how satiated they are—as compensation for the narcissistic injury they suffer at being reduced to subordinate admirers. In this regard, the artist's demanding public may represent the crowd of Freud (1922) and Le Bon regressing to a primitive herd ego. In spite of this, the public is also aware that the artist, in some measure, is symbiotic with it. Protected by the anonymity and enormous distance between itself and its hero-artist, it feels free to exploit that symbiosis by escalating its demands. Unchecked, this can become sadomasochistic; that is, viciously rejecting of what does not gratify it or swooning into a trance of appreciative love when it is temporarily and deliciously satisfied. Finally, this narcissistic, sadomasochistic demandingness of audiences especially upon artist-performers may serve a defensive need: to cover up a sense of their own symbiotic ties to their chosen admired artist.

If the artist and his public represent, then, a special kind of narcissistic relationship, there is a sense in which the performing artist and his audience represent a special kind of group. It is a group which has neither the fight-flight, the dependent or work group basic assumptions described by Bion (1974), nor the cohesive, libidinally identified character considered fundamental by Freud (1922). Instead, the artist and audience may meet once and perhaps never again. The difference between the artist and his audience and the libidinally tied group Freud spoke of, is this: while the audience is united in its appreciative love of the performing artist, the artist works only for the gratification of his narcissism and merely *pretends* to love the audience. This is in stark contrast to Freud's hypothetical group (1922) in which the group leader can actually work and care for the group. Seen in this light, the celebrated, willing suspension of disbelief on the part of the audience also refers to the disbelief (based on reality testing) that there is any true relational or libidinal tie between artist and audience.

In other words, the relationship between artist and audience maintains, in spite of reality testing, two illusions: one, that what is being performed is more than pretense, is somehow really happening; and two, that the artist and audience are somehow emotionally bonded in a way that matters. This is opposed by the counter sense that there is no tie at all between audience and artist, that the relationship is promiscuous, and as soon as one audience has been fully experienced the artist moves on to the next. It is much truer to say that the audience is *used* rather than loved. This is an interesting contrast to Freud's (1922) conception of the group as being an extension of libidinal family dynamics. According to Freud, the sibling's envy of not being loved the most (the favorite) is converted into the illusion that no one is loved more (social justice), with the result that each member of the family (group) feels equal to one another via its common libidinal identification with the father (group leader). In terms of our conception of the artist and audience the process is somewhat reversed. While the illusion is maintained that the group is loved equally (the artist is performing for them *because* he loves them) in reality there is no true libidinal tie between them. Nothing can come of the relationship because it is over as soon as the performance is over.

Summing up, the artist sometimes does seem to carry the messianic hope described by Bion (1975), and sometimes the audience does seem libidinally tied and identified to the leader-artist in a manner depicted by Freud (1922). Yet, it is perhaps more true to say that the group-audience has captured the ego-ideal of the leader-artist than, as Freud pictured it, the leader has captured the ego-ideal of the group. This is one more way of saying that because the artist–audience is a unique kind of dynamic relationship it is also a unique kind of group.

So far, we have been talking about the double bind of the artist in relationship to his creativity and to his audience *prior* to entering therapy. It is important because each of these double binds will come into play, transferentially, as the process of therapy unfolds.

For example, artists often experience a therapeutic double bind in terms of their creativity. How much of it do they reveal? This is hard enough to decide generally. When the artist is an actor (as many of my patients were) there is an added complication and an added double bind. What is the double bind of the actor? Briefly, how to be real in imaginary circumstances; and if one manages that, how does one manage to simultaneously *feel real while pretending* to be someone else? Fine acting suggests this can be done, but that does not mitigate the toll it takes on the actor to produce it nor, especially, the intense long-standing psychical confusion that may precede it. In terms of assessing the degree of talent of the actor, the therapist, short of actually attending a performance—which is a rare occurrence—cannot know. The fact that most actors like most artists, more often than not, are struggling, unrecognized, and unemployed means that there will be an absence of clarifying external professional corroboration. This can be disturbing, countertransferentially, to a therapist who therefore has to operate in the dark on a very important reality issue: he would naturally want to know whether the actor who is banking so much of his life on his talent is banking on an illusion. There is an irony here. The criterion by which professional acting is evaluated by critics is the same criterion by which professional therapists assess *nonacting* in regular patients; that is, by its realness, its moment of truth. The same therapeutic sensitivity to defenses of grandiosity, unrealness in patient productions, can perhaps be applied to the professional efforts of actors—how real it is (this would be so if only we had access to their performances, which, of course, we do not). The creativity of actors in part is a creativity of attempting to resolve the peculiar double bind they find themselves in. The creativity of actors, at least so far as achieving being real in imaginary circumstances, lies in finding a personal way to transform an imaginary situation into something intimate and real. As audience, we can then infer that if an actor has achieved such an impact of powerful immediacy and realness—knowing this has been done in a context which is imaginary in an existential sense—that an effort of concentrated creativity *must* have preceded it. By contrast, in nonartistic patients, equivalent "moments of truth"—that is, a more integrated, cohesive contact with their real self—may indicate *not* creativity but loosening of defenses, strengthened reality testing, and therapeutic working through. The irony is that the true creative core of actor-patients often emerges not in therapy but in performance; and what the therapist cannot see, the therapist cannot be expected to understand.

One particular double bind of artist-patients revolves around the necessity of doing low-level survival work. Artists generally make their art their priority, and therefore seek out marginal jobs (like being a waiter) offering flexible schedules which, initially, they find liberating. They overlook the price they will later pay for their flexibility of hours—the performance of work which in our society is often perceived as humiliating. Since artists are often more narcissistic than the average person, they find themselves as waiters caught in the strange double bind of having to deny their personal, narcissistic needs while constantly pretending to be primarily interested in servicing the narcissistic needs of anonymous, rotating customers. Even the best waiters, in order to perform their job, must do a considerable amount of *pretending*; and even the best actors, as waiters, are scarcely able to bring this off. More important than the fact the conflict is irresolvable (making it a double bind) is that artists, with their greater narcissistic needs, find the work *humiliating*. As therapist to numerous young, struggling unrecognized artist-waiters, I listen to repeated tales of perceived, internalized humiliation at the hands of customers and superiors. Not surprisingly, it sometimes filters down to their nightmares and may appear in the guise of monstrously demanding, overwhelmingly multitudinous customers. One of my patients, a brilliant artist who was hypersensitive to the slightest, perceived rebuff, often dreamed at night of his daytime work as a waiter. He imagined gigantic outdoor cafes, peopled by hundreds of clamoring patrons, situated thousands of feet apart.

Perceptions such as these, common among my artist-waiters, can have a cumulative effect leading to an explosion, real or fantasized, of narcissistic rage. In the movie *Tough Guys*, Burt Lancaster and Kirk Douglas portray a pair of elderly, anachronistic train robbers who are released from prison after decades of incarceration. Their conception of themselves as romantic outlaws is rudely dashed as they reenter the world in the unaccustomed role of powerless senior citizens. In a pivotal scene, Kirk Douglas, trying to support himself as a waiter, suddenly goes berserk at what he perceives as the unbearably humiliating role of gratifying the greedy needs of obnoxious customers. In a defiant rage, he marches through the restaurant in a grotesque mockery of a servile waiter. "Would you like a knife, sir?" (he impales the necktie of the customer to the table with the requested knife). "Some water, Madam?" (pouring a pitcher of water on the woman's head). The movie is broadside comedy, yet the scene hyperbolically expresses a common fantasy of narcissistically wounded artist-waiters, who yearn to turn the tables as an *act of narcissistic retaliation*. This fantasy was actually carried out by one of my patients, Katherine, a beautiful, emotionally volatile, manic actress who was customarily infuriated by her job as a waitress. One day, unable to check her rage at a woman who asked her for one cup of coffee too many, Katherine suddenly took the pot of coffee she was serving customers from and slowly poured it over the woman's expensive fur coat. "Will that be enough coffee?" she asked in a mimicking voice.

The double bind that artists who work as waiters experience and the narcissistic injury that ensues from it is only an exaggeration of what they generally feel while employed in subordinate capacities. There is a curious parallel between the dynamics of performing artist and audience which we have presented, and the dynamics of seller–buyer in our culture—especially, when the product being sold is human services. We explain it this way: the customer, say in a restaurant or hotel, suffers a narcissistic injury to the degree that he fears or becomes paranoid that he has been objectified into a form of narcissistic supply to the seller. The seller is then suspected of having no use for the customer other than exploiting him for narcissistic supplies (typically, money). Realizing this, the seller develops a style of relating that is calculated to reassure the customer—specifically by emphasizing all the narcissistic supplies which the *customer is shortly going to receive*. Much of selling and salesmanship in America revolves around the fine art of assuaging the narcissistic injury inherent in the role of being a customer, someone perceived as an available, tempting source of narcissistic supply (profit), and pursued as such. This is done by a magicianlike trick of diverting the attention, by flattering and trying to whet the narcissistic appetite of the expectant customer. Thus sales- and businesspeople, classically, almost *always* talk enthusiastically about what it is they are going to do for the customer, what benefits they are going to deliver. By contrast, they never talk about what has to be of much greater importance: what they intend to do for themselves, what purely personal, narcissistic benefits they may be hungrily seeking to procure from the cooperation of the customer. It is hardly surprising that in the world of business transactions, service and product benefits have become institutionalized buzz words, in great part because this is what the customer needs to hear.

That there is also an interpersonal defense against narcissistic injury as well as an economic, strategic side can become painfully clear when something goes wrong. The familiar rage seen in people when they feel cheated of the expected service they have paid for (for example, from a waiter in a restaurant or vacation resort) can be viewed as an expression of narcissistic injury upon realization of the true purpose of the transaction: to save as much expense as possible on the customer in order to gain a correspondingly greater profit. In this sense, the rage at not getting their money's worth is not only an indignant reaction to a perceived breach of economic contract but is also, on a deeper level, an attempt to deny and undo a narcissistic injury. Pursuing our parallel between artist–audience and seller–buyer, we might say that the best service like the best acting does not seem manufactured, but appears fresh and spontaneous. Now, since genuine service usually springs from a personal, altruistic, or intimate impulse, it cannot be primarily economic in nature. If it is primarily economic in nature, as all business service must be, on some personal, narcissistic level of the psyche it must eventually ring hollow. From this springs the house-of-cards feeling of possible imminent collapse, the suspicion of phoniness that almost all professional service brings with it. That this must necessarily pertain, given our culture, to even the professional service delivered by a therapist creates well-known resistances. However, when the professional service is primarily economic, and when the suspicion of phoniness is believed to have been proven true, there is an additional narcissistic injury which is defended against. A major defense is denial; specifically, that an injury has not occurred to one's narcissism, but instead there has been a breach of economic contract—one has been cheated. The fact that there is ready at hand an institutionalized outlet for asserting one's economic rights can serve as *a reinforcement for acting out one's denial of narcissistic injury.*

In this sense, *money represents an externalization and projection of perceived unjust depletion or robbing of intrapsychic, narcissistic supplies.*

Artists, perhaps because of their own deep involvement in the double bind of performer–audience dynamics, are especially sensitive to the double bind intrinsic in the process of psychotherapy. As patients they are mistrustful and search uneasily for clues to the real relationship in order to arm themselves against possible future narcissistic injury. Narcissistic patients are especially prone to experiencing the withholding of the true self (therapeutic neutrality) as a narcissistic injury; and artists, because of their own considerable narcissism, are therefore highly sensitive to issues of inauthenticity regarding the process of psychotherapy. They experience the false self (Winnicott 1960) of the therapist as a disturbing narcissistic injury; but, paradoxically, are less sensitive and much more comfortable with their own false self. In other words, *the narcissism of artists in psychotherapy can be used as a defensive mechanism to sustain their own false self.*

Artists in psychotherapy, especially if they are struggling and unrecognized, experience one other double bind. They wish to be evaluated, not on concrete circumstances, but on creative potential. In extreme cases, this may take the form of artists indirectly demanding of their therapists that they be seen, not in the present, but in the future projected light of their to-be-actualized inspiration. To a therapist unfamiliar with artists, this may seem like either shallow narcissism or a request akin to something like a leap of faith on the part of the therapist.

It is a different matter with the artist. The double bind of artistic inspiration is real and is but a special case of the process of creativity. The artist must simultaneously sustain a relationship of intimacy with the deepest sources of his creativity while keeping his eye coolly on the most efficient techniques for marketing and actualizing the implicit vision. Unless one has worked intensively with young, unrecognized artists, it is hard to conceive of the importance which they place on their creative inspiration. Rather than an isolated instance or flash of increased self-esteem, to an artist artistic inspiration can be a vision or possibility of continuous narcissistic supplies. In this sense, the artistic inspiration is more like the dawn of a new relationship—except that it is a narcissistic relationship between creativity and the self. The relationship between the artist and his art, then, is like Freud's (1914) narcissistic object choice: art is chosen because of what it reflects about the artist.

Artistic inspiration differs from other narcissistic object choice relationships inasmuch as the intensely charged narcissistic object, instead of being a person is an impersonal object (art) or process (artistic process). Since this is not often understood, people tend to underrate the sustaining power of artistic inspiration; and to thereby overrate the amount of risk-taking that can go into an artistic project which boasts no visible means of guaranteed payoff in the customary sense. It is a salient characteristic of visionary artistic inspiration—and a source of abiding conflict to artists—that it creates a temporal relationship between the artist and his future success that is essentially internal without manifest props; and that thereby the corresponding reality testing, to a great extent, must be similarly internal.

If artists are so implicated in double binds, as we suggest, what of double bind strategies and techniques to treat them? In our view, double bind therapists who vigorously approach the therapeutic situation as a field to be conquered with the best "strategies" (Haley 1958) will at most achieve symptom relief and behavioristic manipulation; but will have difficulty facilitating enduring structural, intrapsychic, interpersonal, or developmental change.

To return to our original definition of the double bind in psychotherapy: we differ from Gregory Bateson (Bateson et al. 1956) who conceived the double bind as arising from a nexus of paradoxical mixed messages and conflicting levels of communication. Instead, we view the therapeutic double bind as originating from a conflict of incompatible levels of intimacy; specifically, the (unspoken of) conflict between professional technique and intimacy. Accordingly, we see the double bind as intrinsic to the process of psychotherapy, and best handled with empathic understanding and philosophical acceptance.

Richard Feynman, the great particle physicist (1985), said that at the heart of quantum mechanics was a paradox—running counter to any commonsense notion of reality—that has consistently baffled the greatest of minds, including his own. To have even a chance of understanding nature, warned Feynman, required a mind that could be content, could coexist with a thoroughly noncommonsensical world. It may be that in the tiny universe of therapy and analysis, a comparable sacrifice is called for. In our opinion, the good therapist, on some level, knows that the discrepancy between restrained, self-censoring professionalism (no matter how empathically delivered), and continuous, intimate self-disclosure, with nothing held back, is too great to be smoothly, simply resolved. He does not pretend to have outsmarted, conquered, and turned to his therapeutic advantage, the double bind in psychotherapy. He does not boast of "sharpening" the paradox in the hope of achieving a new therapeutic paradox (Jackson and Haley 1963). Neither does he deny or dismiss it nor offer variants of pat answers such as, "You give me the power." Instead, he softens the paradox, while upholding both ends of a paradox he intuitively understands is both necessary and one he will have to live with. So he steers as best he can between the two poles, technique and intimacy, knowing that, in our culture anyway, there is no apparent, true counterpoint in sight, but only a kind of philosophical, stoic acceptance (in the spirit of Richard Feynman) that may be the closest we are going to come to therapeutic wisdom.

2
Yesterday's Narcissism

Early Hopes

What happens when the artist's creative self, which can feel magical at times, gets deflated? The crash can be enormous.

Katherine, the emotionally volatile, manic actress who acted out her rage at having to be a waitress by pouring coffee on a customer's coat, is just one of numerous examples. How far down she had come can be measured by comparing her with the ebullient twenty-year-old, arriving from upstate New York, with a fiery ambition to succeed as a dramatic stage actress. Manhattan was the place to be with its inner world of Off and Off-Off Broadway, showcase plays, theatrical agents, workshops, acting classes, and near infinity of opportunities for artistic exploration, indulgence, cultivation, and self-improvement. With her flowing red hair, startling good looks, and seemingly effortless ability to emote, she would use what she had and do what she had to do to satisfy her longing to act. And at twenty, with energy and dreams to burn, it did not seem that difficult to wait tables, take classes, go to auditions or faceless cattle calls, hunt for agents, hobnob with aspiring as well as established actors and playwrights, live packed into a small studio apartment with one or more roommates, and experiment with assorted and replaceable boyfriends.

It was no hardship at twenty to spend hours composing thank you, reminder postcards to promising agents and interested playwrights she had encountered; to sometimes spend days idling on a Manhattan movie set so that she could appear for a few brief, unspoken seconds as a crowd scene extra. At twenty she could be proud that soon after arriving in New York she landed a part (nonspeaking) in a featured motion picture headlined by major Hollywood stars, in which, for a fleeting magical second, her solitary face and figure commanded the screen. At twenty, it didn't matter that the problems she had gradually become aware of in her early teens—spells of unexplained irritability, extreme difficulty in concentrating, a willfulness about getting her own way that could erupt into explosive rage whenever she felt significantly opposed, and a growing suspiciousness and bafflement over how to decode even the simplest motives of other people—kept cropping up. Even if it were true that she kept rubbing the right people the wrong way, her high-energy, resilient sociability, abundant talent, and willingness to do almost anything (artistically) for a part, more than compensated for this.

To such a twenty-year-old, brimming with talent, hope, and determination, the future, as she scans the artistic horizon, must seem bright. Perhaps a seasoned clinician, or better, a gifted observer of human nature, who had met her then might have sensed that already she was heading for trouble. Perhaps not. At any rate, in retrospect, twelve years later, when I first met her, it seemed clear that her combination of a shaky sense of self and extraordinary creative neediness was a precarious one, and therefore her chances poor of faring well in the devouring melting pot of the transient artistic subcultures in New York City. By the time I met her, Katherine's youthful bravado had all but evaporated and she was frankly, unashamedly desperate.

innumerable jobs as an extra on Manhattan movie sets, which she justified by the relatively high rate of pay, and perhaps hundreds of callbacks for auditions that somehow did not materialize.

Katherine could never understand why, and as the years and auditions rolled by her sense of agitated puzzlement over whether she was in some mysterious, unconscious way repelling people deepened. She kept brooding over these repeated failures, wondering if there were something "bad" she was doing, and after she met me she pressed me over and over again for the answer, the simple magical formula that would unlock and explain her peculiar behavior.

Of course, I had no such formula. It was easy to see how she might alienate people: she had a hair-trigger temper, an irritability that was always close to the surface, and a mercurial unpredictability that made you never sure what she was going to do next. One moment she could be a poetic Blanche DuBois of poignant suffering, and the next she could unexpectedly lash out at you. The suspiciousness that Katherine had observed in herself as a teenager had hardened into something of a paranoid trend. I never knew what might set her off. She might berate herself for being unglamorously ugly compared to TV commercial beauties. I might point out this wasn't the case (innocently enough I thought), and she could snap, "Don't try and support me that way." Or, she might indicate she urgently needed a new monologue for auditions and, when I took the bait, asking her what kind of monologue she had in mind, demand, "What good does it do for you to know that?"

That was one side of the coin (which I generally did not see until months after the therapy began); the other was the helpless side. She managed to make me feel she really needed me. Once when she made one of her unconscious personally cutting, off-putting remarks (and I must have flinched) she seemed genuinely to panic: "Oh . . . you didn't take that personally did you? Please tell me if I say something offensive. I want you to. I so desperately need your help. . . . " There was the time I checked my answering machine early in the morning, as I always do, and heard the

Yesterday's Narcissism

In our initial telephone contact, prior to our first me[eting,] unexpectedly and timidly asked me—as though it wer[e a large] request—if she could call me by my first name. Whe[n I auto]matically said yes, I could hear an audible sigh of relie[f. Impul]sively, Katherine made that a basis of trust and confide[nce. She] had just backed out of an initial consultation visit wit[h another] therapist because she had denied use of her first name. "[My name] is Dr. _____, not Louise" announced my predecessor [whom she] knew and whose imperious air did indeed leave no d[oubt about] who was going to be in charge).

Katherine could be appealing, then, in a forlorn kin[d of way.] Her pathos was real and ran deep, but she did not [tend to] embellish it with a creative flair I have come to expect f[rom some] patients. They often make dramatically cohesive prese[ntations of] their inner miseries which comparably intelligent, but [less imag]native, patients find difficult to do. And Katherine was [certainly] not dramatic. Twelve years of pounding the theatrical b[oards may] have altered her psyche, but it had left her presence [intact. At] thirty-two, despite a distinct pallor acquired from yea[rs of acting] and working almost exclusively indoors, she was still a[pleasure to] look at with her shoulder-length flowing red hair, ch[iseled fea]tures, and proud, upright bearing.

The Dream Fades

The narrative, however, of herself which Katherin[e shared] in the early sessions was one long litany of maddening [frustration,] accompanied by an enraged almost toxic sense of [her own] personal failure. She spoke breathlessly, usually with [much emo]tion, and sometimes with a flight of ideas that could s[hock me.] Considering that most professionals felt she was a gi[fted young] actress, Katherine had amazingly few credits to show [for twelve] years' labor: a handful of showcase plays for which [she was un]paid, some regional summer stock work in Seattle, [and some] paid work as an understudy to a celebrated Off-Broad[way] strangest of messages recorded in the dead of night: "Oh God, please don't be there . . . please don't live there . . . But I have to talk. . . . "

For about ten minutes Katherine, in a rambling anguished soliloquy, poured out the details of a disturbing fight she had just had moments ago, while waitressing, with her boss. She was terrified she was on the verge of losing her sole means of support by being fired, but she seemed even more terrified she had invaded my sleep with her intrusive panic, and every few minutes pleaded, "Oh please, please don't be there." Since Katherine knew I didn't live in my office, I could only assume that her need and wish for me to be there, to contain her sense of impending fragmentation, made me really seem to be there; which in turn produced a fear of possible retaliation for having woken me up, and the anxiety that I, like her boss, would punish her by abandoning her. So she vigorously denied her need for me to be there (to be woken up) so that I could listen to her, by begging that I not be there.

This insight, if it was one, was small comfort as I replayed her message several times. Her voice, isolated this way on the answering machine, allowed me to hear it in a way I had not heard before. The ordinarily rich intonation, magnified by surges of panic, frightened me, in spite of myself. I began to wonder what could have produced such a sense of agitation and despair. It was not hard to find symptoms in Katherine that were popular in books on psychopathology: signs of paranoid ideation, borderline splitting of the ego, flight of ideas, narcissistic personality, manic mood swings. Yet putting her in one or the other of the available diagnostic categories would not meaningfully have explained her, and worse, would have been of little use to a psychotherapist hoping to help her. Her state of acute dislocation and alienation in Manhattan seemed somehow intrinsic to her artist's lifestyle.

Although I had been a therapist for several years, and had met numerous people who could be conventionally described as narcissistic, paranoid, or borderline, this was my first full blown encounter with the day-to-day rigors of someone really trying to make it as an artist in New York City. That world which the young artist entered—often unfriendly, cold, opportunistic and profit-minded—seemed to be a powerful, added, special ingredient with special conditions setting the artist apart into a group of its own. Furthermore, in addition to the unique double binds characteristic of the artistic life-style, there was the equally unique narcissism inherent in the artistic personality (which I have tried to spell out in the opening chapter). Such special qualities were generally overlooked in the textbooks, which customarily include the artist in psychotherapy as just one of a series of subtypes of narcissistic personality disorders. Yet the more I came to know Katherine (and all the other artists that followed her during the next ten years), the more I came to understand how powerful that combination was: on the one hand, an artistic life-style and subculture in a major urban center so indifferent to the individual needs of the arriving artist as to appear alien; on the other hand, certain narcissistic traits (as I mentioned) peculiar to the artistic temperament and a series of double binds that seemed to regularly evolve from the artistic life-style.

Since much of this was generally passed over in the textbooks I had read or the analytic training I had received, I could initially never be sure whether I was copping a plea in the face of the perceived magnitude of my patient's needs. What I did know was that the more I came to understand Katherine, the more baffled I felt as to how to formulate even minimal treatment goals.

The Last Session

Katherine must have sensed this. After several months of being alternately dramatically needy, off into a chattering withdrawal, or indirectly devaluing, what little patience and hope she had for the therapy began to break down. The devaluing, especially of men, became both acute and uninhibited. Once, when she was discussing auditioning for a role in a Shakespearean play and I had asked her how she felt about the part, she suddenly snapped,

"Shakespeare's a faggot. He can't write parts for women." Although Katherine continued to come to sessions, she made it increasingly clear she was finding therapy a pointless exercise and not helpful. She challenged whether I was the proper therapist for her and, in spite of myself, I noticed I was working much too hard to prove her wrong. There was the time when Katherine, feeling stuck in therapy—as she often did—asked me what she should talk about next, and, taken off guard by the question, I had replied, "Whatever comes to mind." Now this was a classic textbook rote response, which I well knew and which probably contributed to the mechanical, stale way I delivered it. It was apparently the final piece of ammunition and confirmation she needed, because her reaction was truly electric. She looked conjointly amazed, deeply wounded, and wracked with agonizing irony. Her contempt was enormous and complete. Slowly she shook her head, unable to contain her exasperated mockery. She acted as though she had been journeying an incredible distance to find the meaning of life and had just been offered the most unimaginably cosmically dumb answer: "I ... I can't do this anymore ... *whatever comes to mind* (beginning to laugh disgustedly) ... No ... I just can't...."

I admit, had Katherine stopped therapy at that point, the vulnerable part of me would have been relieved, but she was not ready to give up her attachment to me, and I was not ready to give up my commitment to help her in spite of herself. Yet determination and good will were hardly sufficient. Katherine was clearly in a downward spiral, and each time I saw her, she was progressively more agitated, distracted, more rambling, more hopelessly restless and suspicious. She made it clear she was coming to therapy against her wishes, a kind of reluctant prisoner waiting for her freedom, which would come only when I granted her permission to leave. I found myself in one of the unhappiest positions a therapist could be in—someone who has been given the warden-like responsibility of deciding whether to hold or release another person from a significant and binding relationship. No longer was there a question of what is technically called resistance analysis, because the thread of the interpersonal alliance that is used to confront the resistance had been snapped. I had been cast, from the vantage point of her paranoia, in the role of the enemy—someone to be circumvented, manipulated, and if possible conquered. Katherine now acted as though it were taken for granted she would be leaving therapy and began using our sessions as a training ground and springboard for her next therapist.

Of her next therapist, there was only one thing she was sure—the gender. It would be a woman. Her experience with me had convinced her that only a woman could truly understand her. While I did not want to accept this at face value, I told her that if that's what she felt she really needed, I would be willing to serve as a cushion and bridge to her next therapist. Katherine seemed genuinely surprised. She considered it an unduly forgiving and generous offer on my part, but she managed to quickly undermine it. About three weeks later when I took my annual summer vacation, approximately one year after I had first met her, she used the time off to secretly recruit my successor.

There was one last session, upon my return, but it was not to, finally, openly disclose her decision to terminate therapy. Instead, it was one more attempt to devalue all that therapy at my hands, a man's hands, had not done for her. The realization that this was probably the only way she could separate—through rage and contempt—did not thereby soften the blow. She had saved the worst for the last: secret vituperative thoughts about me that she had been harboring for months would now be aired:

"Remember that time I asked you for a glass of water? You couldn't seem to make up your mind whether the glass was clean or dirty. Whether to rinse it or let me drink out of it. It took minutes. I thought (beginning to shake with laughter) my God, if he can't handle a glass of water, how's he *going to handle me!*"

"And why—why do you *hide* behind the door? Why do you always open the door, and then *hide* behind it?"

It was small comfort to remind myself (which I found necessary to do) that the passageway behind the door was so narrow that it would have been impossible to open the door, acknowledge her presence, and then let her in without first being forced to step backwards as I pulled the door open. It was small comfort to retreat to the insight that when the magical self gets deflated—as I had seen in Katherine—the artist can begin to feel robbed of inner resources in a way ordinary people do not experientially understand, and which in turn can reinforce any latent tendencies of paranoia. It was small comfort that in the years to come, I would often observe paranoid trends emerging in artists soon after narcissistic depression. All I knew in that final session was how desperately Katherine wanted to communicate to me her sense of personal failure. That she succeeded beyond her wildest dreams—evoking in me a lingering pain and mystification at a therapy gone awry—she would never know.

Three days later, I received a not surprising message on my answering machine—Katherine's official termination of therapy: "I know I shouldn't be doing it this way on the telephone . . . but this is what I have to do. I'm not coming back anymore. I've found a woman that I really want to work with . . . and I'm going to start seeing her. . . . Thank you for your help . . . I'll send you the money I owe you."

Afterwards, I spent a long time trying to understand what had gone wrong, what I might have done better. One thing that had impressed me about Katherine (and with almost all artists I have worked with) was the low priority she put on relationships that lay outside the sphere of her art. Her primary relationship, where most of her psychic energy seemed to flow, was to her art. This is another way of saying that her real interpersonal relationship was that of performing artist with audience (as I tried to describe in the opening chapter). This can go beyond what Freud called a narcissistic object choice: choosing a person on the basis of qualities that either mirror or enhance desired qualities in oneself. Of course, in the case of artists such as Katherine the narcissistic object choice (which, as I suggest, is the audience) is much more impersonal. It is almost as though, especially for the performing artist, the audience is what really exists and what truly counts, while individual flesh and blood people are, more often than not, relegated to fantasy. This was shown by Katherine, first of all, in her transferential relationship to me: it was not just that she treated me as an extension of her psyche, what self psychologists like to call a selfobject. This was true enough. But what I felt was more fundamental, her real selfobject, was the way that she related, poured seemingly her whole being, into her monologues, her auditions, her acting classes, her unending search for the right audience. So long as she was relating to the object of her art, she seemed so much more animated, genuine, and full bodied than when she was relating to isolated individuals such as myself.

Kohut (1971, 1977), the great theoretician of narcissism, has suggested that the healthy narcissism, which in some measure exists in all people, is a major component in the psyches of all artists, especially great ones. The classic example is Beethoven, who though deaf, could have his music validated and internally echoed within his own self-esteem. Following Kohut, self psychologists have extended the presumed healthy narcissism of great artists like Beethoven to imply a generalized healthy self-esteem functioning in all artistic creativity. What is overlooked is the great expense to other areas of the personality extracted by such artistic self-esteem. In fact, it may be that artists, great or small—just *because* they have achieved relative artistic self-esteem—suffer the oft-described deficits in most noncreative sectors of their personality.

This was certainly true of Katherine. Whatever self-esteem or healthy narcissism she had, and she had precious little, was almost entirely invested in her image of herself as a contemporary artist. By comparison, her relationships with people felt unreal and insubstantial. She had trouble differentiating between acting and real life. Often, she would try to resolve her confusion by attempting to evaluate interpersonal relationships the same way she would evaluate a theatrical performance; that is, on the basis of qualities she found aesthetically satisfying. In this sense, Katherine's string of boyfriends were judged generally by the criterion of their dramatic performance.

Nowhere, was this more in evidence than in Katherine's relationship with Michael, the boyfriend with whom she was mainly involved during the year I knew her. Michael, a generally unemployed, frustrated nightclub comedian worked the tiniest of clubs in New York City. As perceived by Katherine, his relationship with her was, almost literally, one of comedy in exchange for sex; that is, whenever he felt sufficiently sexually needy, he would impulsively come over and endeavor—through what he considered the magic of his stand-up comedy—to charm her into bed. Usually, he succeeded. On the one hand, the fact that this relationship, which had been going on intermittently for the past seven years, had little more to offer than this bizarre barter, enraged Katherine. Yet, on the other hand, she found it irresistibly entertaining. There was one memorable session in which Katherine, with tears rolling down her cheeks at what she found adorable goofiness, recounted joke by joke Michael's newest routine: it revolved around a subway commuter who happens to glance down upon the tracks, notices another commuter who has just fallen down, witnesses an oncoming subway train behead the luckless commuter, then gasps as an emergency team of highly trained microsurgeons carefully sew the commuter's head back on. As a special backup prop for the routine, Michael had constructed a gigantic four-foot facsimile of a cinnamon roll to be stood on while delivering the routine, and—upon receiving the customary heckling—from which to triumphantly shout, "Shut up, you _____, can't you see I'm on a roll?"

For such a person as Katherine, then, who needed so much, who was capable of receiving so little, and who often settled for even less, it seemed as I listened several times to her farewell message that she could only be headed for trouble.

The Will to Survive

The East Village in Manhattan where I have my office is a relatively small enclave where the paths of residents can crisscross numerous times. Since Katherine lived only blocks away from my office, it was more surprising than not that in all the years that passed since she had left therapy, I would bump into her just once. She recognized me first as we approached each other from opposite directions along the same street. Except for a pallor which had deepened together with a new somewhat gaunt look, after three-and-a-half years, she had not appeared to have changed. For about a minute we made small talk, Katherine speaking nervously and with forced cheerfulness. For myself, I wasn't sure how lightly or how seriously to approach what might be (and was) the last time I would ever see her, but finally I said what was on my mind, asking her if she had continued with her therapy. She looked at me curiously before responding: "For a while, I did," then, the old suspiciousness instantly reviving, she snapped, "Why do you ask?" I realized there was nothing more I could do for her, shrugged, muttered something tame about wishing her well, and just hoping she had continued therapy, then prepared to say goodbye. Katherine smiled, and for a single moment came genuinely to life: "You know, I'm *still* acting."

Sixteen years after arriving in New York, a gifted and natural actress, she was still pounding the pavements. With an absence of conventional rewards, almost nonexistent reinforcement, in the face of what must have been alarming demoralization and isolation, she pushed on. I had to wonder what drove her. I present Katherine because she is in some ways prototypical of the young artist arriving in New York. Although she is an extreme, and thereby clear case, she is not uncommon. The odds are substantial against the young artist, even if exceptionally talented, achieving what we call conventional success. The majority of them, including those who do ultimately succeed, spend years enduring a day-to-day regimen of varying, yet predictable disappointment. Katherine's existence, although admittedly harrowing and tortured to the extreme, represents the young, aspiring, contemporary artist in this way: on the one hand, there are generally intense, rather special narcissistic needs intrinsic to their artistic creativity; on the other hand, there is a life-style, a subculture—and if we move far enough up the hierarchy—an industry which, in spite of feeding off these needs, is immune to them. This is not to deny what is called psychic reality and to imply that everything is caused by the life stressors of being an urban artist. Obviously, there is an interaction. It does mean the artist will not respond easily to either quick fix or standard long-term therapies.

The artists presented here are *not* the ones usually presented in the literature or textbooks. There is a very good reason for this. The artist who typically appears in the literature, more often than not, is the artist who has arrived at the private and therefore expensive office of a psychiatrist or psychoanalyst and who, by economic definition, would statistically fall into the group classified as relatively successful. That, however, is not the essential artist who, regardless of talent, for a long time does not succeed. Such youthful artist-patients almost never find their way into the office of a contemporary psychotherapist (again) for the very good reason they cannot afford it. For the same reason I am pretty sure the portrait of the artist as a young patient to be presented here, has yet to be drawn in the literature.

As I mentioned at the beginning of this book, by a quirk of fate, I happened to be working for a small, community agency charging nominal fees, which allowed me my choice and fill of artists. By another quirk of fate, I happened to have been a writer myself, who had struggled for many years prior to coming to New York. Whatever empathy and rapport I had as a psychotherapist was thereby strengthened; whatever natural curiosity there was for the process and inevitable sorrows of being a young contemporary artist (yes, there are joys, but remember these are artists who have to find their way to therapy) was intensified.

So here, then, after some necessary (to me) theoretical reflections and speculations on what I have observed over ten years, is the young artist in New York, as revealed through that most intimate of all lenses: psychotherapy.

innumerable jobs as an extra on Manhattan movie sets, which she justified by the relatively high rate of pay, and perhaps hundreds of callbacks for auditions that somehow did not materialize.

Katherine could never understand why, and as the years and auditions rolled by her sense of agitated puzzlement over whether she was in some mysterious, unconscious way repelling people deepened. She kept brooding over these repeated failures, wondering if there were something "bad" she was doing, and after she met me she pressed me over and over again for the answer, the simple magical formula that would unlock and explain her peculiar behavior.

Of course, I had no such formula. It was easy to see how she might alienate people: she had a hair-trigger temper, an irritability that was always close to the surface, and a mercurial unpredictability that made you never sure what she was going to do next. One moment she could be a poetic Blanche DuBois of poignant suffering, and the next she could unexpectedly lash out at you. The suspiciousness that Katherine had observed in herself as a teenager had hardened into something of a paranoid trend. I never knew what might set her off. She might berate herself for being unglamorously ugly compared to TV commercial beauties. I might point out this wasn't the case (innocently enough I thought), and she could snap, "Don't try and support me that way." Or, she might indicate she urgently needed a new monologue for auditions and, when I took the bait, asking her what kind of monologue she had in mind, demand, "What good does it do for you to know that?"

That was one side of the coin (which I generally did not see until months after the therapy began); the other was the helpless side. She managed to make me feel she really needed me. Once when she made one of her unconscious personally cutting, off-putting remarks (and I must have flinched) she seemed genuinely to panic: "Oh ... you didn't take that personally did you? Please tell me if I say something offensive. I want you to. I so desperately need your help...." There was the time I checked my answering machine early in the morning, as I always do, and heard the

In our initial telephone contact, prior to our first meeting, she unexpectedly and timidly asked me—as though it were a large request—if she could call me by my first name. When I automatically said yes, I could hear an audible sigh of relief. Impulsively, Katherine made that a basis of trust and confided how she had just backed out of an initial consultation visit with another therapist because she had denied use of her first name. "My name is Dr. _____, not Louise" announced my predecessor (whom I knew and whose imperious air did indeed leave no doubt as to who was going to be in charge).

Katherine could be appealing, then, in a forlorn kind of way. Her pathos was real and ran deep, but she did not hesitate to embellish it with a creative flair I have come to expect from artist-patients. They often make dramatically cohesive presentations of their inner miseries which comparably intelligent, but less imaginative, patients find difficult to do. And Katherine was nothing if not dramatic. Twelve years of pounding the theatrical boards may have altered her psyche, but it had left her presence intact. At thirty-two, despite a distinct pallor acquired from years of living and working almost exclusively indoors, she was still arresting to look at with her shoulder-length flowing red hair, chiseled features, and proud, upright bearing.

The Dream Fades

The narrative, however, of herself which Katherine presented in the early sessions was one long litany of maddening frustration accompanied by an enraged almost toxic sense of shame and personal failure. She spoke breathlessly, usually with great emotion, and sometimes with a flight of ideas that could seem manic. Considering that most professionals felt she was a gifted natural actress, Katherine had amazingly few credits to show after twelve years' labor: a handful of showcase plays for which she was not paid, some regional summer stock work in Seattle, one week's paid work as an understudy to a celebrated Off-Broadway actress, strangest of messages recorded in the dead of night: "Oh God, please don't be there ... please don't live there ... But I have to talk...."

For about ten minutes Katherine, in a rambling anguished soliloquy, poured out the details of a disturbing fight she had just had moments ago, while waitressing, with her boss. She was terrified she was on the verge of losing her sole means of support by being fired, but she seemed even more terrified she had invaded my sleep with her intrusive panic, and every few minutes pleaded, "Oh please, please don't be there." Since Katherine knew I didn't live in my office, I could only assume that her need and wish for me to be there, to contain her sense of impending fragmentation, made me really seem to be there; which in turn produced a fear of possible retaliation for having woken me up, and the anxiety that I, like her boss, would punish her by abandoning her. So she vigorously denied her need for me to be there (to be woken up) so that I could listen to her, by begging that I not be there.

This insight, if it was one, was small comfort as I replayed her message several times. Her voice, isolated this way on the answering machine, allowed me to hear it in a way I had not heard before. The ordinarily rich intonation, magnified by surges of panic, frightened me, in spite of myself. I began to wonder what could have produced such a sense of agitation and despair. It was not hard to find symptoms in Katherine that were popular in books on psychopathology: signs of paranoid ideation, borderline splitting of the ego, flight of ideas, narcissistic personality, manic mood swings. Yet putting her in one or the other of the available diagnostic categories would not meaningfully have explained her, and worse, would have been of little use to a psychotherapist hoping to help her. Her state of acute dislocation and alienation in Manhattan seemed somehow intrinsic to her artist's lifestyle.

Although I had been a therapist for several years, and had met numerous people who could be conventionally described as narcissistic, paranoid, or borderline, this was my first full blown encounter with the day-to-day rigors of someone really trying to make it as an artist in New York City. That world which the young artist entered—often unfriendly, cold, opportunistic and profit-minded—seemed to be a powerful, added, special ingredient with special conditions setting the artist apart into a group of its own. Furthermore, in addition to the unique double binds characteristic of the artistic life-style, there was the equally unique narcissism inherent in the artistic personality (which I have tried to spell out in the opening chapter). Such special qualities were generally overlooked in the textbooks, which customarily include the artist in psychotherapy as just one of a series of subtypes of narcissistic personality disorders. Yet the more I came to know Katherine (and all the other artists that followed her during the next ten years), the more I came to understand how powerful that combination was: on the one hand, an artistic life-style and subculture in a major urban center so indifferent to the individual needs of the arriving artist as to appear alien; on the other hand, certain narcissistic traits (as I mentioned) peculiar to the artistic temperament and a series of double binds that seemed to regularly evolve from the artistic life-style.

Since much of this was generally passed over in the textbooks I had read or the analytic training I had received, I could initially never be sure whether I was copping a plea in the face of the perceived magnitude of my patient's needs. What I did know was that the more I came to understand Katherine, the more baffled I felt as to how to formulate even minimal treatment goals.

The Last Session

Katherine must have sensed this. After several months of being alternately dramatically needy, off into a chattering withdrawal, or indirectly devaluing, what little patience and hope she had for the therapy began to break down. The devaluing, especially of men, became both acute and uninhibited. Once, when she was discussing auditioning for a role in a Shakespearean play and I had asked her how she felt about the part, she suddenly snapped,

"Shakespeare's a faggot. He can't write parts for women." Although Katherine continued to come to sessions, she made it increasingly clear she was finding therapy a pointless exercise and not helpful. She challenged whether I was the proper therapist for her and, in spite of myself, I noticed I was working much too hard to prove her wrong. There was the time when Katherine, feeling stuck in therapy—as she often did—asked me what she should talk about next, and, taken off guard by the question, I had replied, "Whatever comes to mind." Now this was a classic textbook rote response, which I well knew and which probably contributed to the mechanical, stale way I delivered it. It was apparently the final piece of ammunition and confirmation she needed, because her reaction was truly electric. She looked conjointly amazed, deeply wounded, and wracked with agonizing irony. Her contempt was enormous and complete. Slowly she shook her head, unable to contain her exasperated mockery. She acted as though she had been journeying an incredible distance to find the meaning of life and had just been offered the most unimaginably cosmically dumb answer: "I . . . I can't do this anymore . . . *whatever comes to mind* (beginning to laugh disgustedly) . . . No . . . I just can't. . . . "

I admit, had Katherine stopped therapy at that point, the vulnerable part of me would have been relieved, but she was not ready to give up her attachment to me, and I was not ready to give up my commitment to help her in spite of herself. Yet determination and good will were hardly sufficient. Katherine was clearly in a downward spiral, and each time I saw her, she was progressively more agitated, distracted, more rambling, more hopelessly restless and suspicious. She made it clear she was coming to therapy against her wishes, a kind of reluctant prisoner waiting for her freedom, which would come only when I granted her permission to leave. I found myself in one of the unhappiest positions a therapist could be in—someone who has been given the warden-like responsibility of deciding whether to hold or release another person from a significant and binding relationship. No longer was there a question of what is technically called resistance analysis, because the thread of the interpersonal alliance that is used to confront the resistance had been snapped. I had been cast, from the vantage point of her paranoia, in the role of the enemy—someone to be circumvented, manipulated, and if possible conquered. Katherine now acted as though it were taken for granted she would be leaving therapy and began using our sessions as a training ground and springboard for her next therapist.

Of her next therapist, there was only one thing she was sure—the gender. It would be a woman. Her experience with me had convinced her that only a woman could truly understand her. While I did not want to accept this at face value, I told her that if that's what she felt she really needed, I would be willing to serve as a cushion and bridge to her next therapist. Katherine seemed genuinely surprised. She considered it an unduly forgiving and generous offer on my part, but she managed to quickly undermine it. About three weeks later when I took my annual summer vacation, approximately one year after I had first met her, she used the time off to secretly recruit my successor.

There was one last session, upon my return, but it was not to, finally, openly disclose her decision to terminate therapy. Instead, it was one more attempt to devalue all that therapy at my hands, a man's hands, had not done for her. The realization that this was probably the only way she could separate—through rage and contempt—did not thereby soften the blow. She had saved the worst for the last: secret vituperative thoughts about me that she had been harboring for months would now be aired:

"Remember that time I asked you for a glass of water? You couldn't seem to make up your mind whether the glass was clean or dirty. Whether to rinse it or let me drink out of it. It took minutes. I thought (beginning to shake with laughter) my God, if he can't handle a glass of water, how's he *going to handle me!*"

"And why—why do you *hide* behind the door? Why do you always open the door, and then *hide* behind it?"

It was small comfort to remind myself (which I found necessary to do) that the passageway behind the door was so narrow that it would have been impossible to open the door, acknowledge her presence, and then let her in without first being forced to step backwards as I pulled the door open. It was small comfort to retreat to the insight that when the magical self gets deflated—as I had seen in Katherine—the artist can begin to feel robbed of inner resources in a way ordinary people do not experientially understand, and which in turn can reinforce any latent tendencies of paranoia. It was small comfort that in the years to come, I would often observe paranoid trends emerging in artists soon after narcissistic depression. All I knew in that final session was how desperately Katherine wanted to communicate to me her sense of personal failure. That she succeeded beyond her wildest dreams—evoking in me a lingering pain and mystification at a therapy gone awry—she would never know.

Three days later, I received a not surprising message on my answering machine—Katherine's official termination of therapy: "I know I shouldn't be doing it this way on the telephone . . . but this is what I have to do. I'm not coming back anymore. I've found a woman that I really want to work with . . . and I'm going to start seeing her. . . . Thank you for your help . . . I'll send you the money I owe you."

Afterwards, I spent a long time trying to understand what had gone wrong, what I might have done better. One thing that had impressed me about Katherine (and with almost all artists I have worked with) was the low priority she put on relationships that lay outside the sphere of her art. Her primary relationship, where most of her psychic energy seemed to flow, was to her art. This is another way of saying that her real interpersonal relationship was that of performing artist with audience (as I tried to describe in the opening chapter). This can go beyond what Freud called a narcissistic object choice: choosing a person on the basis of qualities that either mirror or enhance desired qualities in oneself. Of course, in the case of artists such as Katherine the narcissistic object choice (which, as I suggest, is the audience) is much more impersonal. It is almost as though, especially for the performing artist, the audience is what really exists and what truly counts, while individual flesh and blood people are, more often than not, relegated to fantasy. This was shown by Katherine, first of all, in her transferential relationship to me: it was not just that she treated me as an extension of her psyche, what self psychologists like to call a selfobject. This was true enough. But what I felt was more fundamental, her real selfobject, was the way that she related, poured seemingly her whole being, into her monologues, her auditions, her acting classes, her unending search for the right audience. So long as she was relating to the object of her art, she seemed so much more animated, genuine, and full bodied than when she was relating to isolated individuals such as myself.

Kohut (1971, 1977), the great theoretician of narcissism, has suggested that the healthy narcissism, which in some measure exists in all people, is a major component in the psyches of all artists, especially great ones. The classic example is Beethoven, who though deaf, could have his music validated and internally echoed within his own self-esteem. Following Kohut, self psychologists have extended the presumed healthy narcissism of great artists like Beethoven to imply a generalized healthy self-esteem functioning in all artistic creativity. What is overlooked is the great expense to other areas of the personality extracted by such artistic self-esteem. In fact, it may be that artists, great or small—just *because* they have achieved relative artistic self-esteem—suffer the oft-described deficits in most noncreative sectors of their personality.

This was certainly true of Katherine. Whatever self-esteem or healthy narcissism she had, and she had precious little, was almost entirely invested in her image of herself as a contemporary artist. By comparison, her relationships with people felt unreal and insubstantial. She had trouble differentiating between acting and real life. Often, she would try to resolve her confusion by attempting to evaluate interpersonal relationships the same way she would evaluate a theatrical performance; that is, on the basis of qualities she found aesthetically satisfying. In this sense, Katherine's string of boyfriends were judged generally by the criterion of their dramatic performance.

Nowhere, was this more in evidence than in Katherine's relationship with Michael, the boyfriend with whom she was mainly involved during the year I knew her. Michael, a generally unemployed, frustrated nightclub comedian worked the tiniest of clubs in New York City. As perceived by Katherine, his relationship with her was, almost literally, one of comedy in exchange for sex; that is, whenever he felt sufficiently sexually needy, he would impulsively come over and endeavor—through what he considered the magic of his stand-up comedy—to charm her into bed. Usually, he succeeded. On the one hand, the fact that this relationship, which had been going on intermittently for the past seven years, had little more to offer than this bizarre barter, enraged Katherine. Yet, on the other hand, she found it irresistibly entertaining. There was one memorable session in which Katherine, with tears rolling down her cheeks at what she found adorable goofiness, recounted joke by joke Michael's newest routine: it revolved around a subway commuter who happens to glance down upon the tracks, notices another commuter who has just fallen down, witnesses an oncoming subway train behead the luckless commuter, then gasps as an emergency team of highly trained microsurgeons carefully sew the commuter's head back on. As a special backup prop for the routine, Michael had constructed a gigantic four-foot facsimile of a cinnamon roll to be stood on while delivering the routine, and—upon receiving the customary heckling—from which to triumphantly shout, "Shut up, you _____, can't you see I'm on a roll?"

For such a person as Katherine, then, who needed so much, who was capable of receiving so little, and who often settled for even less, it seemed as I listened several times to her farewell message that she could only be headed for trouble.

The Will to Survive

The East Village in Manhattan where I have my office is a relatively small enclave where the paths of residents can crisscross numerous times. Since Katherine lived only blocks away from my office, it was more surprising than not that in all the years that passed since she had left therapy, I would bump into her just once. She recognized me first as we approached each other from opposite directions along the same street. Except for a pallor which had deepened together with a new somewhat gaunt look, after three-and-a-half years, she had not appeared to have changed. For about a minute we made small talk, Katherine speaking nervously and with forced cheerfulness. For myself, I wasn't sure how lightly or how seriously to approach what might be (and was) the last time I would ever see her, but finally I said what was on my mind, asking her if she had continued with her therapy. She looked at me curiously before responding: "For a while, I did," then, the old suspiciousness instantly reviving, she snapped, "Why do you ask?" I realized there was nothing more I could do for her, shrugged, muttered something tame about wishing her well, and just hoping she had continued therapy, then prepared to say goodbye. Katherine smiled, and for a single moment came genuinely to life: "You know, I'm *still* acting."

Sixteen years after arriving in New York, a gifted and natural actress, she was still pounding the pavements. With an absence of conventional rewards, almost nonexistent reinforcement, in the face of what must have been alarming demoralization and isolation, she pushed on. I had to wonder what drove her. I present Katherine because she is in some ways prototypical of the young artist arriving in New York. Although she is an extreme, and thereby clear case, she is not uncommon. The odds are substantial against the young artist, even if exceptionally talented, achieving what we call conventional success. The majority of them, including those who do ultimately succeed, spend years enduring a day-to-day regimen of varying, yet predictable disappointment. Katherine's existence, although admittedly harrowing and tortured to the extreme, represents the young, aspiring, contemporary artist in this way: on the one hand, there are generally intense, rather special narcissistic needs intrinsic to their artistic creativity; on the other hand, there is a life-style, a subculture—and if we move far enough up the hierarchy—an industry which, in spite of feeding off these needs, is immune to them. This is not to deny what is called psychic reality and to imply that everything is caused by the life stressors of being an urban artist. Obviously, there is an interaction. It does mean the artist will not respond easily to either quick fix or standard long-term therapies.

The artists presented here are *not* the ones usually presented in the literature or textbooks. There is a very good reason for this. The artist who typically appears in the literature, more often than not, is the artist who has arrived at the private and therefore expensive office of a psychiatrist or psychoanalyst and who, by economic definition, would statistically fall into the group classified as relatively successful. That, however, is not the essential artist who, regardless of talent, for a long time does not succeed. Such youthful artist-patients almost never find their way into the office of a contemporary psychotherapist (again) for the very good reason they cannot afford it. For the same reason I am pretty sure the portrait of the artist as a young patient to be presented here, has yet to be drawn in the literature.

As I mentioned at the beginning of this book, by a quirk of fate, I happened to be working for a small, community agency charging nominal fees, which allowed me my choice and fill of artists. By another quirk of fate, I happened to have been a writer myself, who had struggled for many years prior to coming to New York. Whatever empathy and rapport I had as a psychotherapist was thereby strengthened; whatever natural curiosity there was for the process and inevitable sorrows of being a young contemporary artist (yes, there are joys, but remember these are artists who have to find their way to therapy) was intensified.

So here, then, after some necessary (to me) theoretical reflections and speculations on what I have observed over ten years, is the young artist in New York, as revealed through that most intimate of all lenses: psychotherapy.

3
Creative Paranoia

The Third Degree

"I know I'm being tape-recorded." Obviously pleased with his accusation, Dan leaned back in his chair, tilted his head, smiled mischievously, and waited for a rebuttal. He didn't seem to be kidding, but then how could he not be? The question took me by surprise. No patient had ever asked me if I were secretly recording the session. I was fascinated by the novelty of the situation it suggested. I asked Dan why he imagined I should want to tape record him, especially without his permission. The shrugging response implied he was just as puzzled as I was, but the smile, suspiciously, widened. It was clear Dan didn't care how or why he had arrived at his hunch, what mattered was that he knew, somehow, he was onto something. It was also clear that he was continuing to enjoy—almost as though he had just executed the winning move in a game being played out between us—the growing possibility that, perhaps for the first time, he had his therapist on the defensive.

Dan might have been right. Despite the fleeting warning to myself not to fall into the trap of being defensive, I had to continue. If Dan didn't know why I was secretly tape recording him, perhaps he knew *how*. I invited him to identify the site of the camouflaged tape recorder, to even explore the office if he thought it might illuminate the mystery. I felt I was doing this, not in the spirit of challenge, but in the hope of establishing a genuine investigative bond. I really did want to get to the bottom of this.

There is a famous case in psychotherapy in which Robert Lindner (1954) describes his valiant efforts to decipher the magnificently intricate delusion of a particular patient, a physicist, who happened to believe that at times he was living on another planet. Lindner begins the analytic exploration, believing he is dealing with an intriguing but manageable patient who suffers from an equally intriguing but manageable delusion. As the sessions mount up, Lindner notices that far from yielding to his analytic probing, the delusion seems to be prospering. In increasingly finer and richer detail, the patient unfurls the secret workings and inner world of his delusion. The patient has enjoyed amazingly interesting visits to the mysterious planet. Exact astronomical calculations have even been rendered. The patient goes so far as to bring charts and notes to the sessions, each pinpointing a presumably critical checkpoint in the mammoth and daring voyage to the planet. In spite of himself, Lindner discovers he is becoming more absorbed in the mysterious planet than in the patient. He can never hear enough about it, and no matter how much information the patient supplies, Lindner hungers for more. He is restless between sessions, counts the hours or days until he will next see his patient in a way he has never done before.

As he begins to anticipate the next planetary visit it is Lindner, the psychoanalyst, and not his patient, who is nervous, agitated, impatient, and barely able to contain his anxiety over the imminent departure. And it is the patient, the patently delusional physicist, fancying himself a voyager to another world, who has gradually become concerned, solicitous, and downright nurturing to his therapist who curiously and unexpectedly has come to share in the patient's delusion. To more than share, to so monopolize the delusion that, finally, in a memorable role-reversal session the patient invites his psychoanalyst to seat himself in a nearby chair. When Lindner does so, the patient kindly, and therapeutically announces: "It's all false," and goes on to explain how he had made it all up, realized weeks ago it was just a delusion, but did not know how to break the news to his analyst who seemed to now need the delusion more than he did. What follows, according to Lindner, is an eventual dramatic cure of both patient and therapist originating from the cathartic reciprocal insights gained by unconsciously switching roles.

The case is wonderful to read, for professional and layman alike, because it shows, on the one hand, the potentiality of the patient not only to engage his therapist's interest, but to sometimes bewitch him; and on the other hand it graphically reveals what can happen when the sensitivity, empathic receptiveness, and human vulnerability necessary to be a professional precariously go astray.

While my patient, Dan, certainly did manage to fully capture my attention, I never felt lost or bewitched by the paranoid twists and turns that would follow his initial accusation that I was secretly tape-recording him. What I did learn, instead, was the kind of unique theatrical aura, the morbid if riveting charm that could seem to encircle the paranoid mind. Listening to such a patient, a therapist can feel, very unlike an ordinary session, as though a stage were being lighted and a cast of thoroughly unreal but quaintly compelling characters was being trotted out. Listening to such a patient, especially when encountering the unexpected, first unfolding of a true paranoid fantasy, a therapist can experience a peculiar ambivalence. Does he believe or disbelieve the patient? Imagine this analogous situation: someone you think you know, whom you do not believe has demonstrated seriously disordered thinking, suddenly announces he has just witnessed a man in the street armed with a machine gun. It seems impossible that he could fabricate such an astounding statement, so your instincts are naturally to go along with him. Yet simultaneously and just as instinctively, a part of you must shrink from embracing such an alien reality and you ask yourself, "A machine gun—in the street?"

The therapist cannot afford the luxury of expressing this ambivalence. He must hold his response, wait, ponder, and investigate. Dan politely turned down my invitation to confirm his suspicion that I was covertly tape recording him. It was more than enough, it had taken all of his courage, in just our third session, to articulate his accusation. Plainly, he was enjoying the original disarray of my surprised reaction. His grinning air of having won an important advantage over me seemed so gratifying a payoff that he could securely decline comment on all my subsequent, exploratory questions.

It marked a pattern that would recur—try as I might I could never tell when—in the weeks, months, and years to follow. Periodically, out of the blue, whenever he felt ready, or sensed I was available as a possible target, he would point the arrow of a paranoid fantasy directly at me. I might, for example, put a tissue to my nose, sniffling and chilled by a dampness in the air and note Dan, with that slow grin, knowingly nodding; and when nothing ensued, when there was only that apparently delicious pleasure at having caught me in some imagined unsavory act, taking the bait, I would inquire, "Dan, what is it—you're smiling?" On this occasion, after the usual guarded silence, Dan had replied, "You're nose is running. You're wiping it." After reflecting upon this for a few moments, coming up with absolutely nothing, and thereby all the more intrigued, I said simply, "I'm sniffling. You're right. So?" "Well," Dan began, who had become cautiously diplomatic and cagey, "you see, when you take cocaine, you sometimes have a runny nose."

To me it was a rather amazing, if not entirely unprecedented fact that a therapist, prior to a session, should take sufficient cocaine that it would subsequently intrude itself in the course of therapy. I was by this time comfortable and undefensive enough with Dan that I could have welcomed whatever fantasies he entertained as to why I was so motivated. Yet, Dan, as I was to observe time and again, would remain indifferent to my overtures at mutual exploration, and ultimately express ignorance as to the origin of the specific paranoid idea. Despite all my experience as a therapist, it was still a remarkable thing to witness in another human being. That no matter how cognitively incongruous, no matter how at odds with reality, a significant, highly charged belief about another person with whom one is involved in a relationship should be maintained with such unruffled certainty, and nary a nagging, inquisitive afterthought. It seemed obvious to me that such gross cognitive deficits must be the price that the paranoid has to pay in order to purchase some very deep, vitally necessary gratification.

But what is it? In the years to come, there would be many pieces to the puzzle, not only from Dan, but from other troubled young artists. With Dan, three months after I first met him, there occurred an incident that, small as it was, would stay in my mind as a symbol of the patient he was going to become. This was a session scheduled two days before Christmas, perhaps the most potent and meaning-laden holiday for most patients. The session was in the evening. The street leading to my office was relatively unlighted. Dan had arrived uncustomarily early and was sitting in his car parked across the street and about thirty yards ahead of my office. In the back seat, Dan had carefully wrapped a bottle of liquor which he intended to give me, in the course of the session, as a surprise present. He saw me walking up the street. He saw me approach the door of the building leading to my office. Then, so he believes, he saw my head turn slightly to the left, briefly but clearly recognize him sitting alone in the darkened car ninety feet up the street, and (inexplicably and inexcusably) *pretend* not to have seen him.

All of this came out in the session that immediately followed the incident. What impressed me, once again, was the absolute certainty with which Dan had arrived at his conclusion. My best efforts to get him to reconsider his fantasy, the meticulous pains I took to point out the inequity of the lighted building door and the completely darkened interior of the car—making it impossible from a physics standpoint to have recognized him—did not dent, let alone shake his belief. In fact, during the entire session, it was never the question of his belief but only the acknowledgment of my guilt which was at stake. Dan was so sure he had nailed me that he did not bother to hide his pleasure that he had at least furnished proof of my untrustworthiness so dramatic that even I would be compelled to confess.

During that session I became acutely aware that paranoid thoughts, often presented as straightforward, air-tight, deductively arrived at indictments, are really crystallizations and epiphanies that suddenly seize the mind. Epiphanies of what I didn't know. It was part of the crystallizing, paranoid certainty to show no impulse to question the origin of the belief. Such paranoid infallibility, Dan shared. There was no interest in deliberating upon the sentence he had passed upon me. There was just the issue of determining the punishment. "I didn't bring the bottle." Dan smiled hugely as he delivered my punishment. And I had to admit, Dan had been an effective judge. Although I do my best to refrain from accepting holiday gifts from patients, unless it would apparently damage their feelings and our relationship, the thought of a carefully selected Christmas bottle was a warming one. This, however, would be the present that I would never, could never, because of my crime, receive. Over the years, I more than once wondered what the mysterious brand of that taboo bottle had been, whether I would have found it appealing. It was a measure of how artfully he had teased me, how cunningly he had succeeded in whetting my curiosity.

In the months that followed our first session, Dan slowly and cautiously admitted me into his confidence. It was not an easy thing for him to do. Along the way there were certain tests, mainly in the form of sly accusations, which I had to endure. Passing such a test usually meant that I had stood up to, absorbed his accusation and all that it implied, without resorting to angry retaliation: I had neither abandoned, despised, nor devalued him following his attack—all signs he was carefully on the lookout for. As a thera-

CREATIVE PARANOIA   53

pist, it meant I had to be especially on my toes. I could never be sure when Dan was going to spring one of his surprise tests on me. Because of this, paranoia—all other things being equal—adds a strain that does not exist in other therapeutic relationships. Yet, the payoff, if one handles the strain can be rich: the patient takes you into a private, hidden, strange world that can, as I hope to show, be spectacularly interesting.

So I was content in the first few months of therapy with Dan to cultivate a budding, if problematical trust which would enable him to tell me more and more. Dan did. He came into therapy first of all because he was afraid a growing feeling, a welling tension somewhere in his head "was going to explode." He couldn't say what "going to explode" really entailed, but it was clear it had something to do with going crazy. It was also clear that if anything was driving him crazy, it probably had something to do with his job. Dan worked as a messenger for a Manhattan dispatching agency. Originally hired three years ago as just a part-time messenger for Manhattan, he now worked up to sixty hours a week and regularly visited each of the five Metropolitan boroughs. He felt trapped, enraged that he felt trapped, and confused as to how he might have fallen into such a trap. Worse, Dan felt that something "was going on." Not exactly a plot or a conspiracy—"You don't think I'm paranoid, do you?" Dan would, suspiciously, smilingly ask—but he was sure that a few of the dispatchers did not like him and were out to humiliate him. The methods of humiliation were various and tricky. Not tricky enough, though, for Dan not to unravel them. Did they send him to Houston Street with specific instructions to deliver an important manilla envelope to the *fourteenth* floor and did Dan, after triple-checking the address, discover there *was* no fourteenth floor? Well, he knew what they were doing. Did they signal him on the special beeper he was required to wear, and when he answered it, did Mike, the Irish dispatcher—who *knew* he was half Armenian and half French— suddenly exclaim, "Danny-boy!" Once again, he knew what they were doing (I could not resist at this point asking just *what* they were doing). And Dan earnestly explained: "Don't you see? They know I am Armenian but they pretend I am Irish so that they can call me "Danny-boy... Danny-*BOY!*"

I now saw the light. In the world of the blue-collar, macho dispatchers who exercised a blend of belittlement, random abuse, and punitive control to enforce their precarious authority, Dan somehow felt his individual manhood was being personally singled out and slighted. So traumatic was this perception that, try as I might, I could not help him to put it in a more impersonal and objective perspective. They were trying to break him down, to humiliate him by making him fail the test, to show that he was something far less than a man, that he was in fact a Danny-*BOY*. He was certain of this. As certain as he had been that I had secretly tape-recorded him and that I had maliciously pretended not to have seen him in his parked car so as to also humiliate him.

As I got to know him better, I learned some of the reasons why he was so sensitive on the subject of his manhood. At the age of twenty-five, he had never been able to achieve even a single erection while lying in bed with a woman. He was tall, athletically stocky, dark-skinned with an appealing, cherubic face, so there were lots of opportunities and he had tried on various occasions. He stopped trying when no longer able to endure the shame of failure. One woman, in particular, who was very infatuated and very sexually frustrated with his repeated impotence, wondered aloud if the problem might be that he was really homosexual.

Dan was certain, once again, that he was not. He pointed to the fact that all his sexual fantasies concerned women, that in the privacy and safety of his bedroom in the company of his favorite girlie magazines he had no trouble achieving either an erection or an orgasm. It must mean something. On the other hand, he was acutely aware, since his late teens, that he was painfully homophobic. Men followed him in the street, stared at him at beaches, he believed, and sometimes mistook him for a homosexual. People would giggle at him behind his back when he passed by in public places or even sometimes be so brazen as to erupt into explosive laughter. He could never figure out why, but he was sure of it. Eyes are the most popular organ; they appear everywhere and dominate the paranoid fantasy. Dan was certain, when he was fifteen, that eyes were watching him, eyes that he could not seem to escape. Taking his courage in his hands, he confided in his mother, who promptly referred him to a psychiatrist. For six months, Dan cautiously spelled out his fantasy of being stared at. The psychiatrist, an elderly, kindly man (according to Dan) patiently listened and stressed, throughout, the normalcy of such adolescent fears. Dan left feeling comforted but wondering why the psychiatrist had been staring at him so much.

In the microcosm of psychotherapy, there are milestones or breakthroughs as such. About a year after I had first met him, and shortly after Dan had revealed his initial teenage encounter with a psychiatrist, I noticed a disturbing change in my erstwhile shy, if slyly rebellious, patient. Instead of accusing me, and then surreptitiously glancing away, Dan was now boldly trying to stare me down. It was an uncomfortable position for a therapist to be in. Increasingly, I became self-conscious of my own eyes, for the first time wondering where and just how I should look. I waited and hoped that Dan would eventually comment on what was happening between us, something that was steadily growing more painful. I was reluctant to introduce the subject myself, fearing that if it were difficult for me, it would be much more so for him.

When Dan didn't, when his frightened staring continued and even worsened, I felt I had no choice but to take the initiative. It was easier said than done. Never before had I experienced a patient persistently trying to stare me down. Unsure how to proceed, afraid I might make a serious mistake in a delicate situation for which no guiding technique has been laid down, I did what I usually do: I spoke from the heart as plainly, tactfully, and honestly as I could. There was an unfortunate situation that seemed to have arisen between us, I said. From my perspective, it seemed that Dan was staring at me more and more boldly. At times it seemed as though Dan were even trying to stare me down. Of course, I might be all wrong, but that is how it appeared to me. Yet, I could imagine, on the other hand, that is also how it might seem to Dan. I recalled how vividly he had recently been presenting in therapy the powerful and upsetting impact created by the eyes of strange men. Could it be the naturalistic, face-to-face setting of psychoanalytic psychotherapy, in which therapist and patient were more or less forced to continually exchange glances, was recreating an old trauma? I told him I could imagine how such a misunderstanding could arise. I confirmed that I was indeed carefully and intently looking at him, waiting, scrutinizing, trying to understand more deeply whatever his response might be. While that was my job, I did not think and did not intend it to mean otherwise—that is, to be an intrusive, penetrating, and possibly degrading stare. But perhaps Dan thought differently, thought that my look was a stare, and my intent to understand was really just another ploy to humiliate him. Such a misunderstanding, if it had arisen, was unfortunate but, surely, here was the place to discuss it. I ended by earnestly inviting Dan to let the chips fall where they may, and candidly speak his mind.

In Philip Roth's novel, *My Life as a Man* (1970) there is a memorable scene between the author and his fictive analyst. At a key beginning point in the analysis, the analyst says what under any other circumstances, the author points out, would be an ordinary sentence. Yet, the few brief words have a bombshell effect. They stun Roth, leaving an impression that in dramatic punch can rival the greatest sentences in world literature. Roth's point, of course, is not how brilliant the analyst was but how powerful the effect of therapy can be, especially at critical junctures. In terms of my patient, Dan, and in the context of the year of therapy that had passed between us, it was fair to say that the words I had just uttered, at least visibly, affected him the most. Following my invitation to let the chips fall where they may and candidly speak his mind, Dan looked startled, blank-eyed, frightened, and nearly immobilized. My impulse was to rush in and assist him, to get him off the hook that I had put him on, but I checked it and waited. After some very tense moments, and some painful hesitation, Dan, looking at the floor, began to speak. It was true, he said. Yes. He had been feeling for a long time that I was looking at him, staring at him. For a long time it had intimidated him, it had made him respond by looking away, but he had grown tired of that. Why shouldn't I look away at least once in a while? He would secretly test it out. He would stare boldly at me. He would not break his stare until I looked away. If I did not look away, it would be proof I was trying to stare him down. Why, he did not know. So we talked for about forty-five minutes about eyes, his eyes and my eyes, and what were behind them. I pointed out that as I became aware of what was developing, I had in fact been looking away more often than in past sessions, but that in face-to-face psychotherapy, there really was nowhere else to look but at him.

Dan nodded. He had been listening and speaking, with greater concentration that I had ever seen him, occasionally pausing for a short reverielike state—perhaps to process all that was happening. When it was over, he was manifestly and audibly relieved. Never in his life had he even commented upon, let alone entered into such an extended discussion with a man whom he believed was rudely staring at him. It felt different, it felt good. It was, in fact, in Dan's words, "our best session." He was smiling when he left, not happy, but happier than I had known him to be.

Dan, the Would-Be Rock Star

Partly because of this, Dan took me further into his inner world. His inner world was a very musical one. He was a singer, a song writer, a guitarist, an originator of a contemporary rock band that circulated along the small club circuit and could even boast a tiny but growing following. But most of all he was a singer, something he had felt called to naturally and very early. As early as seven years of age. Dan remembers finding or fabricating a small, toy-sized microphone with which he would—yelling and jumping around, already play-acting at being a future rock star—audition before his mother's bedroom mirror. When he was nine, he added a guitar, as backup to his singing, fumbling, finding, eventually picking out his first chord without any help or formal instruction. He wrote his first song when he was twelve and by the time he was fourteen, suffering from increasingly severe bouts of depression, he could ease the loneliness by serenading himself in the privacy of his bedroom, on his favorite guitar, with songs both old and new. The new were rock, most of which had been written by himself, but the old were love songs, sentimental oldies from the fifties and sixties. He had learned them listening by the side of his mother, as she played them over and over again on the antique-looking phonograph set on the coffee table in the living room, usually after dinner.

He was very close to his mother. He could remember, as far back as when he was five years old, stubbornly walking behind her, determined to go wherever she went, following her from room to room. According to a family photograph (which Dan showed me) she was a gracefully built, poetic-looking woman who was depicted cuddling a puppy in her arms as she stared, apparently distracted, off into the distance. Highly artistic, she would regularly retreat into her private studio in order to paint or sculpt. Dan would count the hours until she returned, occasionally throwing a tantrum to accelerate her arrival.

When he was seven, an event occurred which Dan believed was highly important, with possible long-standing traumatic consequences for him. He either overheard or was told directly by his mother one of her greatest family secrets. When he grew older, he would use it repeatedly to explain and rationalize to himself his mother's own artistic self-absorption and bouts of depression—a phenomenon he was increasingly disturbed by and sensitized to. Dan came to believe that his mother's family secret, revealed to him when he was seven, contained the key to all her future depression. The secret was this: when his mother was herself nine years old, attracted by an uncharacteristic noise, she had ventured to the attic where she discovered her own mother, who had just hung herself from an overhead beam using venetian blind cords severed from the bedroom windows. From that point on, as Dan would hear over and over again, his mother—who considered herself a happy child up until the age of nine, although she can remember nothing of that period of her life—would be permanently altered and forever melancholy.

For Dan, who was seven, his trauma did not consist in simply hearing for the first time his mother's family secret. It went beyond that. It touched on his much too intense, symbiotic identification with his mother. It triggered in him a preoccupation and morbid curiosity to know what death was, an obsession that (in retrospect, according to Dan) could have been life threatening. He was referring to a strange period, lasting about a year until he was eight, when he would periodically experiment in play-acting, though possibly dangerous, autostrangulation fantasies. Lying prone on his bed, with either a length of strong twine to simulate the venetian blind cords used by his grandmother or the belt from his trousers, he would progressively strangle himself. He thought he had to know what it felt like to hang himself, had to know in order to participate in the experience of his grandmother, in order to understand the impact it had on his nine-year-old mother whose life was forever changed. As an adult, Dan did not remember if or what he discovered as a seven-year-old. He thinks he might have passed out on more than one occasion. Perhaps he might have been even naked some or most of the time, but does not remember any sexual excitations.

When he was sixteen, his mother died unexpectedly of a heart attack. He remembers the ensuing months as a kind of numb, blank stretch of time during which he did not feel anything in particular. There was his father, though, who used to come into his room in the early morning hours, to console, or more probably to be consoled by his son. Dan liked his father but did not understand him. For example, when his father came into his room in the morning, it was often to invite him to a nearby court for a game of handball. Didn't he understand that having to play handball, a sport he despised, with his father, with whom he barely talked anyway, on the heels of his beloved mother's death, would be the last thing on earth to comfort him? His father, a wealthy, very successful importer, who seemed to live for his career, was always doing things like that. He would make significant gestures, designed to manifest and cement contact with his son's world, which Dan, invariably, found self-serving and phony. No, he would derive little comfort from his father, and wasn't about to give him any.

Drugs were another story, and when his friends, who were all experimenting with a variety of chemicals, urged him to join them, he accepted. Dan was sixteen at the time, the memory of his mother's heart attack still traumatically alive, and he needed another friend besides music. So he plunged into drugs, progressing rapidly from alcohol, marijuana, and cocaine to the more potent psychedelics, especially LSD. For a period of six years, he roamed from one drug of choice to another, becoming increasingly dependent, until he had to stop.

Two things made him stop: a bad experience and a bad trip. The bad experience involved cocaine and the dealer friend who supplied it. Dan, now a freshman at New York University, had been using and sharing cocaine with his friends, steadily, for about a year. From the very first time he had started taking drugs, he had been unable to sample a taste, and then stop. He had to go until he was "wasted." So, when he took cocaine, usually on a party night or a weekend fraternity-brothers bash, he would binge, and the binge could last for days. Dan and his friends always found it easy to designate a given night, "party night." It would begin with Dan staying up all night, drinking alcohol, followed by cocaine, being unable to come down and go to sleep, being unable to stop. It would spill over into the next day. Whatever Dan had to do, he was unable to do. If it was work, he would call in sick. If it was school, he would cut classes.

When the crashes became more catastrophic and the depressive aftermaths more lingering, he went to Narcotics Anonymous (NA). It was a small meeting place situated on the second floor of a building located in Manhattan's Bowery. Dan had chosen the first group he could find, and he had not chosen wisely. He found himself shoulder to shoulder, closeted with a group of very tough street characters. By and large, these were people who had done hard time in prison, who were numbered regularly among the chronically homeless, and who, in the classic parlance of the rehab counsellor, had "bottomed out." Dan, rich boy of a rich family, despite his likability, his easy charm, fun-loving musicality, and adolescent image of counterculture, drug-rock-rebel, clearly did not fit in. His fascination with the novelty of his new peers quickly rubbed off. Always painfully self-conscious, Dan became aware of new eyes, and new hostile stares. He felt pressured to keep step with the approved lingo, terminology, mores, and rules of conduct deemed appropriate for the recovered cocaine addict. If he slipped (and Dan slipped frequently), there would always be at least one wise guy, some hard case, to say I told you so. After one such horrendous lapse followed by a fresh attempt to sincerely recover, Dan remembered an especially vivid rebuke from someone to whom he had confided his slip, and whom he had mistakenly considered a reliable, sympathetic friend: "You know, rich boy, I'm not surprised. As a matter of fact, I bet ten dollars you'd never make it."

Dan moved on, changing rehab centers as often as he had previously changed his drug of choice. Eventually, he settled on a semisophisticated, semi-Yuppie Alcoholics Anonymous group located near Columbia University. It was a near perfect choice. He loved the camaraderie, the ceremonious medals awarded to new members achieving recognized milestones of sobriety: there was one for the first thirty days of abstinence, and there was a very special one for the first ninety days of sobriety. Most of all he loved the attention. Dan was forever counting down days of sobriety, hoping and dreaming he would one day reach the mythical milestone of ninety days sobriety. He never did. He would regularly relapse, regularly be shame-ridden, and regularly be welcomed back with loving arms whenever he summoned the courage to confess his slip and enthusiastically resolve to "do another ninety." When a year of this had gone by, Dan realized he might be an addict.

He was not receptive to rehabilitation, but he was certainly receptive to trauma, and the bad experience which contributed to his giving up drugs was highly traumatic.

Dan was nineteen years old, living in a tastefully furnished apartment on the Upper West Side, completely paid for by his father. News travels fast along the drug grapevine, and his amiable accessibility, his willingness to share on the spot whatever drug he happened to be using with whomever he happened to be talking to, made him an attractive oasis for a steady stream of friends, acquaintances, or plain hangers-on. It wasn't that Dan didn't mind the intrusiveness or that it didn't make him paranoid—it did. It was just that he didn't know how to stop it, nor how to say no. As an example, he was regularly visited at all hours of the night or early morning by the prostitute who lived two floors below him. The visits had nothing to do with sex (a source of constant paranoid worry to Dan) but were to share drugs, exchange drugs, buy drugs, sell drugs, or simply have company while one crashed. Six years later, when I first met him, he was still being woken up by the same prostitute, still unable to say no.

It was in this context, when anyone could knock on his door at almost any hour of the night, that Dan's bad experience occurred. It began with a knocking on his door at 4 A.M. Dan was startled, not so much by the hour, by the knocking, but by the desperate urgency of the sound. He remembers being frightened looking through the peephole. It was Bill, whom he considered his good friend, and the dealer who sold him most of the cocaine he used. But something was wrong. Bill looked pale, disheveled, sweating. He had obviously been running. Dan remembers looking down the hallway nervously to see if someone were actually pursuing his friend. In Bill's right hand was a brown paper bag. All he said was, "Here, take this, please, and get rid of it for me." There was uncustomary but overwhelming gravity in his voice as he handed the bag to Dan, who, again unable to say no, took it, and then ran down the stairway. Instinctively, Dan knew the contents of the brown paper bag; what he didn't dream of was the enormous size of the contents. It was a bag of cocaine with a street value of at least $5000, a quantity about ten times bigger than Dan had ever seen. In the parlance of the user, "Get rid of it" meant only one thing, flush it down the toilet. But how could he? It was like flushing some precious, life-sustaining substance down the toilet. It seemed too easy to stash it, tell Bill he had gotten rid of it, then use it as he pleased.

It was at this point that Dan's paranoia kicked in in a way it never had before. It was early Friday morning. Dan cut his NYU classes and for the next three days paced around his apartment in a gathering agitation. At least a dozen times, he sat himself on the bathroom floor, his hands shaking as he suspended the bag of cocaine precariously above the toilet bowl. Each time he was unable to do it. But what if he didn't and he was somehow caught with his stash? Would he be arrested and sent to a federal penitentiary? Could they do that, blame him for just helping his friend? The more Dan thought about it, what at first seemed inconceivable, by degrees, became possible, and then another certainty.

He began wondering who had been chasing his friend and where he had run off to. He had expected to hear from Bill by at least Friday night to make sure Dan had done what he had been entrusted to do. When Saturday morning came and there had been no contact whatsoever from Bill, Dan was certain he had been arrested. That was the only explanation. But he would soon receive a telephone call from jail from his friend. After all, he was probably Bill's best friend and he would be the logical candidate to arrange bail.

When Sunday morning came and he had still not heard from Bill, Dan now knew that it was not the narcotics agents who had gotten to Bill. It was someone from the drug world, a criminal. No, maybe the mob. Dan shuddered. The idea of someone cold-bloodedly perpetrating a crime, especially the crime of hurting another person, was so alien to his essentially passive, gentle nature that it gave Dan a certain perverse, vicarious thrill. Martin Scorsese's *Mean Streets*, depicting neighborhood gangsterism, had always been one of his all-time favorite movies. It was a different story, though, if the mob were after your friend, if the life they brazenly planned to violate were as close as that to your own. Dan now knew they had gotten to his friend, had beaten him up, perhaps badly. The call that he would get would not be from jail, it would be from the hospital. He was certain of that.

When Monday morning came, and there was still no contact

from Bill, Dan knew why. He had been murdered. It was clear what he had to do. He flushed $5000 of cocaine down the toilet, thus destroying the evidence. His one remaining, but very great fear was that somehow he would be linked to Bill. What if they had followed him to his apartment at 4 A.M. Friday morning? What if there had been a face hidden in the corridor darkness witnessing the transfer of the brown bag from Bill to him? He would have to lay low and take his chances. He would have to act inconspicuous, as though nothing was wrong, to throw them off, just in case there was still a seed of doubt in their minds.

So Dan went to all of his classes at NYU that Monday afternoon pretending not to be in the great danger he was certain he was in. When he came home that evening there was a message on his answering machine from Bill: "Just wondering if you did what I asked you to. Please get back to me." Dan realized at once that Bill was hoping, but not expecting, that he had not flushed $5000 down the toilet. Feeling great relief—he had been hyperventilating throughout the day—he rushed to telephone Bill. Yes, he informed him, feeling bad for his disappointed friend, he had done exactly what he had been told to do. It was gone. Bill sighed: "I guess I just got a little paranoid Friday morning. That's all. But things are cool now."

For Dan, things would not ever be cool so far as cocaine was concerned. He never took the drug again. Listening to all this, I suddenly understood what it was, how potent the paranoid projection had been when Dan accused me of sniffling in a session because of cocaine use. I also realized just how remarkably effective a trauma can be: in its capacity as a negative reinforcer, something which causes someone to "bottom out," it can accomplish, seemingly in hours, what years of therapy or rehabilitation centers often cannot—separate an addict from his addiction. It was positive, healthy, that Dan never took cocaine after that episode. But the intensity of that weekend, the manner in which he fell so completely under the spell of his paranoia (despite its powerful precipitating catalyst), was, I felt, a bad sign and a warning of things to come.

A BAD TRIP WITH THE GRATEFUL DEAD

It was an even worse sign when Dan revealed to me in graphic detail the dimension of "the bad trip" which he now credits with having permanently freed him of all drugs. The bad trip occurred during his attendance at a Grateful Dead rock concert. It was ironic, according to Dan, that something so bad came out of something so beautiful. The Grateful Dead was one of the supreme loves and passions of his life. Until now, when Dan began telling me how his bad trip came about, The Grateful Dead had been nothing to me but another cult rock group. How wrong I was. Dan told me how The Grateful Dead, for those who experienced and truly appreciated them, was *the* band, the ultimate in psychedelic music. Nothing else could compare with it.

Once started on the subject, like a fanatical tour guide, Dan could not stop. Their history seemed his history, and it poured out of him. How they were like a pure culture of the best of the sixties' spirit preserved and transplanted into the eighties. How people, groupies, literally scheduled their lives so as to synchronize with the itinerary of the band's tour stops. How, even beyond that, there were hard-core "dead-heads," people who had grown up with the band in the sixties and did nothing with their lives *except* follow them around, waiting for the next performance. How the spirit that radiated from the people in attendance at one of their concerts, was the most communally loving, freest, and most peacefully blissful he had ever known.

Of course Dan had succeeded in arousing my curiosity even more forcefully than he had when he first teased me with the gift that would never be given. It was no surprise, therefore, that when one Sunday evening I fortuitously made my initial live contact with The Grateful Dead groupies, I was genuinely excited. At least on a visual level, they were everything Dan had said they were. They were milling around outside Madison Square Garden and in the underpasses of Pennsylvania Station, following a Grateful Dead concert, and they indeed looked like no one else. They seemed collectively stoned but they did not look or behave like other stoned people. They were homeless—sometimes congregating in vans or travel buses, trying to eke out a minimal living by selling childlike, organically grown products—but they did not look like any of the other homeless who populate the streets of Manhattan. In an entirely different way, their astonishing psychedelic life-style seemed as unforgettably alien-looking, insulated, and colonylike as the more sociologically celebrated Amish.

Out of all the rich "dead-head" mores Dan had so enthusiastically tutored me in, as a clinician, naturally one stood out. It was the fact, the tradition, that if you really wanted to participate in a Grateful Dead concert you had to be psychedelically tripping at the time. And Dan really wanted to participate. From the age of seventeen when he first tried acid, until he was twenty-two and had last tried it, Dan estimated he had taken well over one hundred LSD trips, not to speak of a variety of other hallucinogenics. Many of them he had taken while in attendance at a Grateful Dead concert. He could never remember a time when he had attended a Grateful Dead concert and not taken LSD.

While he had experienced what he would term "bad trips" before, they had never been enough to interrupt or deter the flow of LSD trips. This particular LSD trip, originating during a Grateful Dead concert—which Dan credits with putting a permanent stop to all his drug taking—was something utterly different. It was, according to Dan, a trauma second only to the death of his mother, in terms of the impact it registered on his life. After more than one hundred relatively satisfying LSD trips, he was unprepared for his final trip. That it occurred in an arena, in the midst of which he felt spiritually, blissfully secure and musically fortified, rendered him doubly unprepared. Dan thinks, but is not sure, that his ultimate bad trip was connected with the evening preceding the concert. He had just been with his girl friend, the one who was both seriously infatuated and sexually frustrated over his prolonged impotence, who had wondered aloud if Dan might be a closet homosexual.

What Dan does know is that his girl friend's roundabout accusation had been ringing in his brain just prior to taking the

LSD. Upon hearing this, it seemed clear to me that if there had to be a villain for his bad trip, Dan preferred it to be his girl friend and not his sacrosanct Grateful Dead.

He does not remember much of the first twelve hours of his last trip. Just that it was the most painful, upsetting experience of his life. A friend who accompanied him to the concert stayed with him the next three days, as a guide to help bring him down. He refused to be taken to the hospital, fearing that it would be reported to his father who would no doubt retaliate by severing his allowance, which would leave him helpless.

What made an indelible impression upon Dan concerning his bad trip, was not the first few days, as terrible as they were. It was what followed. For about three weeks Dan felt completely disoriented. He was unable to recognize familiar faces, unable to form a coherent picture of who he was, unable to recall his name. Six months after the incident, he suffered regularly from long spells of memory lapse, cognitive confusion, and a horrible sense that his brain no longer functioned properly. One year later, after he had returned to NYU and resumed some facsimile of normal day-to-day living, he was convinced he would never be competent at anything that required clear thinking.

In my office, as Dan told me this, his fingers would sometimes grope in the air in front of his face, as though he were trying to geometrically represent the damage that had been rendered to his brain. Perhaps, he thought, if I could see, picture what he was saying, I might have a better chance of understanding it, and helping him. He still, right up until this day, has momentary flashbacks of the gruesome experience. At times, he would surprise me by announcing, "I'm having a flashback—I think." When asked to describe it, he would shake his head: "I can't."

I asked Dan whether, during or after the experience, he had consulted a medical doctor. He nodded yes. Two doctors and one neurologist. All told him they could find nothing organically wrong with his brain. I myself could not tell what impact, if any, his consumption of LSD had had on the etiology of his paranoia. Certainly he manifested paranoid ideation, but to what extent it had existed before his sixteenth birthday when he first started taking drugs, and to what extent it was brought on or brought out by the actual chemical consumption, I couldn't tell. Of course, he must have already been considerably paranoid by the time he was fifteen, when he was deeply troubled by the fear that strange men were continually and suspiciously staring at him. But outside of his paranoid thought disorder, I could see no other sign of cognitive dysfunction.

This was now two years after I had first met Dan. He had settled into the rhythm of therapy and, in his paranoid, testing way, trusted me about as much as he could trust anyone. He no longer suffered from the anxiety that something in his head "was going to explode." He had made an uneasy peace with the dispatchers and was better able to differentiate between unpleasant but general bantering and personal slights. He seemed less paranoid, although his paranoia was always close to the surface, ready to be activated by the slightest pressure. Much of the therapy during the first two years was to help Dan cope, to ensure that such slight pressures stayed slight and did not get out of hand. It was never easy. There was always either a real crisis or a pseudocrisis looming on the horizon. His favorite motto, designed to capture and guarantee my attention, was "Dan's in trouble."

But he did seem to be slowly and progressively getting into less and less trouble. It was an encouraging sign. And even though Dan stubbornly clung to his belief that he would never be able to achieve anything in the straight world above the messenger level, he continued to pour more and more of his free time energy into his musical ambitions. He wrote more songs, rehearsed more, practiced his singing, showed unaccustomed initiative in trying to land his band more bookings. He even added a new hobby: he became a street performer in Washington Square Park or Central Park, when the weather would allow it, offering himself as a lead singer in whatever trio would have him, even overcoming his paranoid shyness (which was at its height) when the hat for donations was passed through the crowd.

And the crowd, whether in the street, or in the confines of a small club, loved Dan, who could really sing. This was brought home to me in yet one more memorable session, when Dan, bolder than ever before, took me by surprise. He had made a tape, consisting of a medley of romantic ballads from the fifties and sixties which he had listened to on his mother's phonograph as a child. Sitting on a park bench in Washington Square Park, Dan had sung directly into a simple microphone hooked up to a tape-recording machine. Bill, still his friend although no longer his cocaine supplier, played backup guitar. More excited and pleased than I had ever seen him, Dan had brought the tape which he held in his hand. Could he play it, for just a few minutes, on my answering machine which sat on a table to Dan's right? It was an offer, somehow, that I couldn't refuse. Although I had known him for two years, although tales of his music had constantly filled my office, I had not once heard him sing.

As a therapist it is a novel and sometimes moving experience, to switch from the customary verbal mode and suddenly make direct sensuous contact with the artistry of your patient. The metamorphosis from patient to artist can seem instantaneous and magical. For the ten minutes that I listened to him, Dan sang beautifully, his voice a pure tenor, filled with self-confidence, feeling, and effortless self-control. The song that I remember was *Love Is a Many Splendored Thing*. There was no doubt Dan put his entire heart and soul into that one, performing it à la the young Eddie Fisher. And it was poignant. Dan, who felt profoundly impaired in his capacity to be sexually intimate with a woman, somehow, in his imagination, was able to artistically—and convincingly—transform himself into a Great Lover.

The two-year milestone in Dan's therapy was important not only because of what had preceded it, but because of what followed it. Looking back on it, I don't think I was especially overconfident or considered myself to be on top of things. From the very first moment I laid eyes on Dan, I sensed how crisis-prone, how fragile he was, and on what precarious footing any momentary gains we achieved would rest. The fact there had been a growing number of such gains which had accumulated over the past two years, that no major crisis had ensued, had not made me complacently less uneasy, but it had given me, in retrospect, a false hope that I could therapeutically handle and contain whatever came up.

Approximately two years after I accepted him as a patient, Dan was to show me just how wrong I had been. Originally, he came into therapy complaining that something was going "to explode in his head," fearing he might lose his mind. Two years later, he appeared to have been a prophet. Dan crossed over the line. The line is hard to define. It is analogous to the imaginary line that is said to exist for alcoholics, which once crossed holds irreversible consequences. In the case of Dan, the line separated what were for him periodic paranoid distortions from a full-blown, clinical psychotic episode. If there is any single prognostic sign in the case of the paranoid it is when the familiar plot and cast of characters, constituting the conspiracy, begin to exponentially multiply. Where previously there were one or two principal tormentors, there are now many. They come from everywhere and they appear everywhere.

It seems safe to say *whenever the paranoid plot mushrooms the illness is growing.*

And the impact upon the patient is unmistakable. Where before, there was an aura of malicious playfulness, a gamelike quality—so that as therapist you could never be sure just what the patient was feeling—there was now an unprecedented earnestness and depth of emotion. Dan appeared in more pain, confusion, and genuine terror than I had ever seen him or I had ever heard him tell me about. Where before the panic would continue for hours, perhaps days, as in the incident when Bill asked him to get rid of a $5000 bag of cocaine, it now lasted approximately two months. Gone was Dan's sly smile, his style of indirect, demure accusation. In its place, were a perception of crisis so real, a sense of urgency so alive, and a state of psychical alarm so convincing that at times I half expected someone to come barging into the office in pursuit of him. While before, no matter how badly or how persecuted he felt, Dan and I could count on relief being somewhere around the corner, it was different now. Dan had the hopeless air of a doomed man sentenced to die. He wore a grim hangdog look, like a spy in an enemy camp who has been flushed out and knows the game is up. Where previously he was the cunningly hidden undercover agent, it was he who was now dangerously visible, surrounded everywhere by multiplying, hostile eyes. Dan's hopelessness infected me, and I became uncomfortably aware of an incipient countertransferential panic. Not being a psychiatrist, and therefore not at all used to working (and not wanting to work) with drug therapy, I had encountered relatively few extended, psychotic episodes. Compounding my dilemma was the fact Dan, ever since his last traumatic LSD trip, was absolutely adamant and paranoid on the subject of any drug taking. My attempts to get him to consider exploring a psychiatric consultation, just in case medication might be helpful, were stubbornly resisted.

One thing was on my side. After two years of willingly taking, and apparently passing, his paranoid tests, I had managed to win his trust. Dan had been steadily admitting me into his inner world. When that inner world turned actively psychotic, Dan had even more reason (and the necessary trust) to let me in. It was an opportunity I must have been waiting for, because I seized upon it.

The episode began inauspiciously. Dan, responding to his beeper, had checked in with Mike, the Irish dispatcher, who greeted him: "Danny-boy. You're the best and I need you." After two years of therapy, Dan had spent a number of sessions discussing his suspicions of the appellation "Danny-boy," his conclusion that the word *boy* contained a hidden message and slur on his manhood. He was still unable to shake his suspicions, but he was better prepared for it and able to live with it. This time, however, something new was added. Mike had called him "the best" and even said "I need you." At first, Dan was thrilled. It was a vote of confidence, the recognition from macho Mike that Dan hungered for, and for about a day he felt blissfully accepted. The next morning mistrust, suspiciousness, and paranoia set in. It could not be possible that Dan was "the best." He was a lowly messenger, and although he killed himself to do a praiseworthy job, there were far more efficient messengers than he was. There was one more thing: Mike never used expressions like "I need you"; he was much too macho. Therefore, he could not have been serious. Dan concluded that Mike had been toying with him, perhaps making fun of his manhood again. But why, what had he done wrong?

All that afternoon, Dan thought about it, searching for the clue, the missing puzzle piece that would explain it. About six o'clock in the evening, just before he was scheduled to sign off, he found what he was looking for. Dan had gone to a Wall Street firm to pick up a new package plus a signed receipt for a delivery he had made the same morning. The delivery in the morning had been a bag containing a sheaf of bearer bonds. The purpose of Dan waiting until evening to collect the signed receipt was to enable the company to accurately tabulate the immense number of bonds. On his way home that same evening, Dan kept studying and restudying the signed receipt. He had a hunch, an uneasy feeling that something was wrong. The confirmation came when he happened to glance at the serial numbers in the upper righthand corner of the signed receipt. Dan was startled to discover that the very last numeral, a five—he was certain he remembered it from the morning—had been changed to a six! Holding the receipt inches from his face, he could still make out faint erasure marks. There was no doubt the number had been changed. But what did it mean?

Dan spent a sleepless night attempting to answer the question. When he went to work in the morning he felt more drained, panicky, and paranoid than he had for years. He was sure something bad was going to happen.

The first thing he noticed was that Mike, the dispatcher, seemed strangely aloof. Not only did he not call him Danny-boy, nor explain why he had teasingly referred to him as "the best," but he absolutely and uncharacteristically frowned at him. Dan knew it was yet another message. By now he was becoming increasingly

CREATIVE PARANOIA 73

dizzy and overwhelmed with the flood of recent messages. Yet, he continued to stay vigilant, on guard, because that was the best way to protect himself. He had learned that long ago and once again it paid off. Late in the afternoon, feeling so agitated and exhausted he was considering excusing himself from work, something he never did, the answer—spectacularly—came to him. It was perhaps the most dramatic crystallization and epiphany he had experienced: *someone had switched the bag.* Of course. There could be no other explanation for switching the number. But why had someone switched the bag? The answer again seemed inexorable: in order to steal the bearer bonds.

But who had done this? It seemed less important to Dan, at first, to determine the identity of the thief than to make sure that Mike realized the innocence of Dan. After all, Dan had been inadvertently involved in the switching of the bag. It seemed logical, then, to keep careful watch over Mike, to notice even the slightest hint that he might be suspecting Dan. When three days of such intensive surveillance produced nothing, Dan felt greatly relieved; then, as was his pattern, he became suspicious. Mike was too smart not to have spotted the difference in the serial numbers on the receipt that went out (which he always checked) with the serial numbers on the signed receipt that came back (which he would check even more thoroughly). Therefore, Mike knew that the bag of bearer bonds had been stolen, had to know, yet he was behaving as though nothing had gone wrong, was once again being friendly with Dan, once again calling him "the best." "The best!" Suddenly the diabolical irony all along hidden in the phrase revealed itself to Dan and he knew: *it was Mike who had stolen the bearer bonds and it was Mike, because of his contempt for Dan, who was setting him up to take the blame.*

It is the nature of the paranoid episode that there is no going back partly because there are no boundaries to guide one: it is like falling into a bottomless, expanding chaos where there are only suspicions, certainties, then more self-doubts which never seem to end. In session after session, Dan appeared cowed, desperate, and hopeless. Where before there had been small crises which had usually been aborted, circumscribed, or successfully managed, now there was an unbroken state of perpetual alarm. Dan now saw faces everywhere that were watching him. It was only a matter of time before one of them stepped out of the crowd, to claim him, to get him. It could be a federal agent or it could be someone from the mob. He was being trailed by certain cars that had been assigned to follow him everywhere. He purchased extra locks for the door and windows of his apartment, and doubly bolted everything in the morning and before he went to sleep.

To no avail. Dan became certain that someone, somehow, was slipping into his room after he left for work in the morning—probably to search for conclusively incriminating evidence that he had stolen the bearer bonds. He would lay his own trap. He took a pair of penny loafers and placed them a few feet behind the front door, at a well-calculated 45-degree angle. Not suspecting this, the intruder who was prying open his front door, would have to automatically bang into them. If the loafers were in a new position upon Dan's return, he would know. Carefully, so as not to spring his own trap himself, Dan eased himself through the front door, which he opened narrowly and rushed to inspect the loafers. They were there—but at a 60-degree angle and *not* the 45-degree angle he had deliberately contrived.

He could stand it no longer. Armed with his own conclusive evidence, Dan went to his father. He must have forcefully pleaded his case, or else just worried his father with the desperateness of his mental state, because his father, normally a prudent man, promptly called the family lawyer, who in turn telephoned the vice president of the firm Dan worked for and left a curt message: "Dan thinks he's being set up."

The magical arm of his father lending support, via the family lawyer, appeared to work wonders for Dan. More than immensely relieved, he was elated, positively thrilled. To whomever was trying to harm him, he had delivered, finally, a powerful message, and a master counterstroke. Naturally, he was bursting with curiosity to discover the reaction of Mike, the man who was behind all this, when news of the family lawyer's warning phone call filtered to his ears. For two days, he bided his time, deriving secret, malicious pleasure from his anticipation of Mike's imminent dismay; knowing, for once, he had the upper hand.

Dan's comeuppance was inevitable and swift. He was delivering a package in the Columbus Circle area when he became aware that he was being followed by a very pretty, red-haired woman. In fact, being chased. Catching him by the arm, the woman, short of breath, exclaimed that she knew him. Wasn't he the one who had sung so beautifully in Washington Square Park? Yes, she was certain she had seen him perform in a trio several times over the past month. She smiled warmly, encouragingly, sexily. Dan smelled a trap. He rarely scanned the faces of the crowd assembled to hear him perform, but he was certain he had never seen this woman before. What was her name? Mary, she said slowly. Dan nodded as though in acknowledgment, accepted her business card, and scrutinized her as she glided away.

"Don't you get it?" Dan smiled ruefully after presenting the encounter in laborious detail. "No," I answered, not bothering to hide my (as usual) complete mystification, "I don't." Dan settled back in his chair, obviously energized. He loved this part of therapy, posing riddles to me, hoping to stump me, and then triumphantly offering the solution: "M, Mary . . . M, Mike. Do you see?"

Now I did. Dan meant that Mike had somehow gotten Mary to seductively tantalize Dan. The secret message was that Mike knew that Dan was impotent with women, and it was sent as a retaliation for Dan's brazen enlistment of the family lawyer. What mattered most to me, though, was not the correctness of this insight, nor the specific content of Dan's most recent suspicion. It was the manner, the style in which Dan had delivered it. Gone was the air of panicky, perpetual crisis. In its place was the familiar (and therefore welcome) provocatively sly, malicious playfulness. I breathed a sigh of relief. Dan was finally coming out of the woods and returning to his old self.

For the full two months the episode lasted, although I had been anxiously bracing myself almost from the start, Dan had not once expressed a suspicion that I was part of the conspiracy out to destroy him. It was a measure, I suppose, of the trust I had accumulated over the past two years through passing his tests or managing to elude his traps. I had paid my dues. Since Dan was too terrified to consider a psychiatric consultation, much less psychotropic medication, it meant I had to work, essentially, without backup. Apart from experience and acquired resourcefulness, all I really had was his trust.

I decided to use that trust. Paranoia, by its nature, must be a very lonely preoccupation. Therefore, if you are permitted by the paranoid to enter his most secret fantasies—that is, if you are not too threatening, if you have mastered the delicate art of applying the right dosage of intimacy at the right time—then you can be not only a relief, but a welcome companion. Although Robert Lindner, by his own admission, crossed over the line and became overidentified with the delusion of his patient, I believe it was the extraordinary vulnerability, openness, and acceptance he displayed which won him the trust of his patient. And it was this, more than anything else, which eventuated a cure.

As I mentioned at the beginning of this chapter, I never did feel I got lost in the material. But I was long fascinated and mightily curious. My strategy, which arose kind of spontaneously on the heels of my enthusiasm, was this: to join him as a paranoid companion, but a more benevolent, saner one. I would accompany him wherever he wanted to go, investigate every puzzle he wanted to investigate, track down every clue, ferret out every hidden message. I would stop short only at the moment, the threshold of reaching a mad conclusion. My strategy was always to subtly shift emphasis to a contrary, more benign perspective, to introduce to his growing and already huge conspiratorial cast another set of equally interesting but less malign characters.

And Dan loved this. He accepted my views as opposing but not adversarial, well-intentioned although clearly wrong. Winning me over, finding the irrefutable evidence that would force me to his side, became a tantalizing challenge. That I was so open to each piece of evidence, allowed Dan in his mind to consider me a fair jury, one he had a chance of convincing. I was glad Dan was so motivated to convert me, because he could not do so unless he took me deeper into his inner world.

Becoming acquainted with the twists and turns of that labyrinthine world, gave me the traveler's knowledge I required. The fact that his pivotal paranoid ideas of reference were really dramatic epiphanies and crystallizations meant that there would be many missing cognitive and logical links. The fact that paranoids insist, as a necessary defense, on the air-tight logic of their suspicions meant, on the one hand, they felt obliged to demonstrate overwhelmingly supportive evidence, and, on the other hand (because of numerous missing links), would be unable to do so. It was therefore relatively easy to back Dan up, to begin by taking all his facts at face value, and then tactfully, gradually pointing out inevitable gross inconsistencies in his own account. My hope was to thereby plant a few seeds of doubt that would erode the rigid certainty that armors the paranoid's world. My method was never to focus on the actual ideas of reference, which were too traumatically frightening to be uprooted, but to shift emphasis to the antecedent *process* leading up to the traumatic event. Thus, for example, I rarely discussed those dramatic revelations when Dan realized that the bag had been switched, that it was Mike who had stolen it, and it was Mike who was setting up Dan. Instead, I would focus on *how* the bag had been switched and stolen, and *why* Mike had chosen to set Dan up. I would count on Dan being naturally curious as to the motivation behind these events, while simultaneously having to admit he was at a loss as how to explain them.

In a sense, I was trying to introduce a greatly simplified model of the psychoanalytic historical method into Dan's paranoid world. Did Dan want to describe those stunning moments when he realized that Mike was setting him up or that the 60-degree rotation of his penny loafers proved the presence of an unseen intruder? I was glad to accommodate him, although not for long: soon I would be working *backwards* inviting Dan to speculate on the intriguing motivation that had to underlie such spectacular behavior. It was not hard to arouse his curiosity and he was willing to join me on just about whatever investigation I proposed. What on earth had induced Mike to steal the bearer bonds, I mused. Time and time again I reminded Dan that for two years he had been steadily caricaturing Mike as a "fun-loving, party animal." How had Mike been transformed, in the style of Michael Corleone in *The Godfather*, into a master criminal? How had someone been able to undo all the locks in his apartment and leave not a single trace save a 15-degree increase of rotation in his penny loafers? How had Mike suborned Mary? Had he placed an ad in the *Times*, interviewed a group of women until he found the right one, then carefully coached her in the precise art of pursuing, teasing, belittling, and mocking Dan?

There were no answers to any of these questions. They were all mysteries to Dan. They troubled and tantalized him. On occasion he would lapse into genuine meditative silences. At other times, the absurdity of his own conclusions would loom so large even from his own delusional vantage point, that he would be forced to ironically, derisively retract his erstwhile certainty: "So you think maybe Mike didn't set me up?" In the paranoid world of iron certainty, such self-doubt was welcome and refreshing. I would use it to reinforce a central interpretation I would make to Dan based on my perception of paranoia as (among other things) a lonely state in which a person (usually extraordinarily fragile) simultaneously dreads and longs for intimacy.

Much of the monsters and torturers that infest the paranoid mind could be understood as a delusional form of negative attention, that is, they keep the paranoid company by being so diabolically interesting, but, because of their evil, they never threaten him with the greater danger of intimacy. Accordingly, my central interpretation to Dan, whenever he seemed poised on the brink of admitting a key idea might be wrong (e.g., that Mike had solicited Mary to mock him) was this: "Doesn't it seem that Mike would have had to have gone to a great deal of trouble to have gotten Mary to do that? Do you really think you're that *important* to Mike?" My interpretation was based on my belief that the paranoid's delusion of persecution is also a delusion of grandeur. By

CREATIVE PARANOIA   79

saying what I did, I hoped to deflate the underlying grandiosity of paranoid thinking. And whenever I made this interpretation to Dan, it did seem to make him stop and think. It was not that he was taking it in, just that he was considering it. Yet, the simple fact that Dan could even consider that one of his major revelations might have indeed been an error, that he might have been acting paranoid, seemed to greatly relieve him, to give him more mental breathing room and restore him to a saner part of himself.

Although Dan's paranoid episode as such completely petered out after two months, the crisis in his therapy had been reached several weeks earlier. After Dan "discovered," via his penny loafer trap, that his apartment was being entered, he decided he had reached the end of the line. It was only a question of time before he was murdered. Desperate, and utterly exhausted, Dan felt he couldn't and wouldn't wait for that to happen. He had to escape. His way out came in yet another exhilarating flash which he announced to me in the following session. He was going to commit suicide, probably by an overdose of sleeping pills. He already had the pills. Now he just had to summon the courage.

This was the moment in the entire two years I had known Dan that I felt most panicky. Once again I tried to persuade him to at least consider a psychiatric consultation and once again he refused. I decided to extend the strategy I had been using, with some success, to his suicidal fantasies. I pointed out that not once in the past two years had he mentioned a single suicidal thought, and I invited him to explain to me the process by which he had unexpectedly arrived at such a momentous decision. Dan welcomed the opportunity. He told me it was a matter of time before he would be murdered, and that he could no longer stand it. Pacing back and forth for many hours in his apartment he suddenly heard a voice, or a whisper, inside his head or outside it. The voice told him that the way out, the only way out, was to commit suicide. I asked whose voice was it. Dan said he thought it was his grandmother's, the one who had hung herself in the attic, and whom Dan had never seen, but had always wanted to see.

It was at this point, that Dan enthusiastically mentioned the movie *Ghost*, which he had just seen. The movie, which is about a man who is murdered but who comes back as a devoted ghost to watch over and protect the woman he loved, had made a deep impression on him. It seemed to serve as a romantic, if bizarre justification for the suicide he was planning. I then told Dan that by coincidence (which was true) I happened to have seen the same movie, and, seeing that he was pleased, I asked if he imagined that afterlife might be something like the movie pictured. Dan said he didn't know if there were ghosts in the afterlife resembling those depicted in the movie, but he definitely believed in spirits. He then added, as though it lent logical support to his intended action, that he was a firm believer in reincarnation. I told him I had encountered a number of people who believed in reincarnation, but I had never met one who also believed in suicide. I then added that I was sure that people who believed in reincarnation—just because they so valued each stage of life and wanted to make it as precious as they could—would be *opposed* to suicide. For a few moments, Dan seemed to think this over, then shrugging, he returned to the movie. At least that showed there could be such a thing as an afterlife, an afterlife that could not possibly be any worse than his present life on earth.

I then asked Dan to imagine for me, in as much detail as he could, how he pictured the afterlife that would follow his suicide. I could see it was something he had never remotely dreamt of, and the chance to discuss this with another human being for the first time was an adventure he relished.

For about a week, we discussed the afterworld that Dan imagined (actually invented) lay waiting for him. I tried hard to avoid the adversarial role. I listened, asked questions, and offered lines of inquiry. Only when Dan had fully mapped out the territory of the afterworld and had populated it with the spirits he envisioned did I offer my alternative world view. I suggested as gently and subtly as I could that if each spirit carried the traits of its mortal ancestor, as Dan insisted, then each spirit should more or less resemble, in personality, the character of its ancestor. Dan nodded agreement. Then, it followed, I continued, that there would be friendly spirits, just as there are friendly people here, and nasty ones, ones like Mike who would tease and belittle him. I paused. Dan had been listening intently and was waiting for me to continue. "What makes you think you'd be any better off there than here?" He was silent. "At least here, you have someone you trust. Me."

I had counted on capturing Dan's artistic imagination with our joint flight into the afterworld, and it had. Dan seemed diverted, entertained, perhaps grateful to have had my prolonged company in the thick of his suicidal fantasies. As a gift to me (he later told me), because he clearly perceived I was on the side of his living and not dying, he went home that same evening and flushed his sleeping pills down the toilet. It was the first and the last suicidal fantasy he ever mentioned.

When I look back on all that happened, it is hard to tell just what had caused the termination of his paranoid episode. Certainly, some of it, or much of it, could have been spontaneous remission. I am sure the fact that he found the courage, born of desperation, to enlist his powerful father's help—who, taking pity on his distraught son, immediately responded—definitely tranquilized his panic. I also feel his acceptance of me as a steadfast companion, one who was allowed to function as a corrective, benign guide, introduced into his paranoid fantasies a potent therapeutic catalyst for change.

Restored to his former self, Dan stayed in therapy for another year, at which time his father relocated to the Midwest. He took Dan with him. Wanting to rescue his son from the dreariness of being a messenger (to which he attributed his madness), he found a small record shop which he purchased for his son. The idea was that Dan would have a cushy managerial job that would enable him to comfortably pursue the musical, rock star dreams he had never abandoned. Dan packed his guitar and countless songs, said goodbye to me and to therapy, and happily left New York City.

Dan had remained drug-free for the three years he had been in therapy, had managed most crises in his crisis-prone life except the major one, but had gotten through a potentially life-threatening paranoid episode relatively unscathed. That was something. But if I had to assess the most important benefit he derived from therapy it was this: he was appreciably, at the end of the third year, much calmer, more centered, and less panicky than he had ever been; he was less prone to paranoid thoughts, could nip them in the bud more quickly, and could retrieve himself from their consequences more efficiently. The years of work we had done together of constant exploration, examination, and reconsideration of his paranoid fantasies had not only enabled him to trust me, but more importantly, it had earned him his own trust. Dan seemed to have acquired, at last, a self-therapizing function to counteract his pathological tendency toward paranoid ideation. It was probable he would always be vulnerable to paranoid distortion, but at least he seemed considerably less vulnerable. I wished I could have done more. I would have loved to have put a dent in the impotency that paralyzed him and helped him with his first intimate relationship with a woman, a fantasy he repeatedly voiced in therapy, but it was not to be.

I didn't hear from Dan after he moved with his father to the Midwest. I often thought about him, though, and wondered what had happened to him. Especially whenever I heard the name The Grateful Dead, or the nostalgic, balladic strains of *Love Is a Many Splendored Thing*. And, whenever there was mention of an exciting, emerging rock star, I was naturally curious (hopeful really) to see if it were Dan.

It would have been hard not to have learned something about paranoia, among other things, from working with Dan. What surprised me was how often the themes, strategies, and underlying dynamics which governed Dan's convoluted thinking would pop up (in various degrees) in other patients, both artist and nonartist. It was not that artists were necessarily more prone to paranoia than other patients; what was different were the preconditions for the emergence of the syndrome, and, especially, the style and flavor of paranoid thinking which is distinctive with artists. Unlike other patients, who, stemming from a whole host of narcissistic injuries, may respond with a paranoid defense, the artist often is abnormally sensitive to narcissistic injury in just one area: his creative persona. When an artist feels creatively dried up, blocked, thwarted, unrecognized, invalidated or just dead the loss can seem as huge, the hole in the psyche as gaping, as when, for example, a nonartist is suddenly abandoned by someone they love. On these occasions, if there is a latent paranoia in the artist, it may be triggered or aggravated by the narcissistic injury to his creative self. If paranoid thinking, in such instances, does truly emerge it is to be expected the superior imaginative resources of the artist, somehow, will come into play. Although paranoid thinking by its nature (Shapiro 1965, 1981) is rigidly restricted and narrowly focused, there is still room for inventiveness. Time and again as I listened to Dan—although he certainly had his favorite plot and his favorite cast—I had the impression I was in the company of a clever play doctor, someone who could alter scenes and characters according to his whim. Because I was thereby sensitized to the possibility of creativity being defensively used by artists such as Dan, I began to look for it in the paranoid productions of other (admittedly less imaginative) nonartistic patients. What I found (as I hope to show) was this: that in *all* paranoia there is an intrinsic element of necessary theatricality, a desire to fictively reinvent the self, and a driving insistence on controlling and rearranging the details of one's inner world that can be reminiscent of the author's celebrated omniscient point of view.

Let me begin with Dan, with some lessons I learned repeatedly from him. The paranoid searches, and does not stop searching, until he finds the evidence he needs to confirm a troublesome suspicion. Threat so dominates the psychic picture that it must never be forgotten, it must always be attended to. Because the paranoid is already attuned by his internal perception and certainty of imminent threat, when it does appear, in no matter how slight a form, it can be traumatic. Dan was frightened of men long before he became aware they were staring at him. When he did notice that certain men were looking at him, it was therefore more than frightening, it was terrifying. It makes perfect sense, given the preconditions. Imagine, for example, that you are convinced there is something terribly wrong or odd about you and are fearful, because of it, you are about to be held up to public ridicule. Couple this with the fact that sooner or later someone, by the laws of probability, is going to begin to stare rudely, threateningly, mockingly, intrusively, or sexually at you. We then have the precondition for a minitrauma, one that can foster and grow unless there is a corrective feedback. Unfortunately, the paranoid rarely has access to such self-corrective, therapeutic feedback.

As David Shapiro (1965) has shown, the paranoid style of thinking manifests itself in a narrowed focus and unrelenting vigilance which in turn creates a fertile breeding ground for suspicious thought. Also, according to Shapiro, because it is so obsessed with being narrowly self-consistent and seemingly logical, paranoid thinking is noncontextual. He means that because paranoid thinking is so predominantly fixated on looking for and finding clues to confirm nagging suspicions, it misses everything else: and everything else, by definition, must include all those positive, warm, emotional signs that should contradict, modulate, or at least put into a more balanced perspective and context those original, attention-getting, threatening, negative signs. Calling paranoid thinking noncontextual is a theoretically interesting way, therefore, of summing up the obvious but important fact that paranoid thinking is distorted.

Suppose, we take this idea of paranoid thinking being noncontextually distorted and consider it in the light of Freud's original theory of catharsis and abreaction as a way of understanding and treating hysterical phenomena (1896). According to Freud, in normal thinking when pathological repression is not a factor, there is an automatic tendency for potentially disturbing affects, through cognitive associative linkage, to drain off. In other words, a potentially upsetting emotional experience, by getting associated with analogous thoughts and feelings, becomes less concentrated, becomes cognitively worked through, and thereby less potent. By contrast, when an experience, for example, an unacceptable sexual arousal in a young girl, is so traumatic as to be effectively repressed, the reverse conditions are set up: the upsetting experience, just because it is barred from conscious, cognitive working through, grows more upsetting until it becomes what we call traumatic.

Freud explained the conversion symptoms of hysteria seen in the young Victorian women he treated as the disguised ramifications of such pent-up, repressed trauma. Freud's cure was to psychoanalytically make contact with the original traumatic memory, bring it to consciousness, achieve the necessary catharsis, and thereby abreact (drain off) the painful affect. When Freud turned to paranoia (1911b), his thinking had advanced to the point where he did not require as explanation a single traumatic experience which had been repressed. In place of the specific trauma were unacceptable homosexual impulses that were repressed primarily through the primitive defense mechanism of projection. Paranoid fantasies, accordingly, were explained by Freud as being the pathological symptoms of repressed homosexual impulses.

Now let's look at the idea of paranoid thinking being a noncontextual distortion. Remember, this means that the abnormally narrowed focus of paranoid thinking precludes the broader context of variable thought and feeling appropriate to real life experience. If this were so (and my experience suggests Shapiro is right) it would follow that the opportunity to drain off potentially upsetting experiences through normal cognitive associative linkage (which Freud considered so important) would also be missing. But it would not be missing as a consequence of the operation of any Freudian repression. It would be missing, would simply follow from the formal nature of paranoid thinking which prohibits normal cognitive, associative working through as a result of its restrictive, noncontextual character. This means, however, that paranoia may be a *cognitive trauma* which is caused by just this noncontextual character. This does not deny that there may in addition be an underlying repressed trauma which is causative in the etiology of paranoia. What it does suggest is that there does not *have* to be such a repressed trauma: the formal characteristics of paranoid restricted thinking are sufficient *in themselves* to develop the traumatic distortions we associate with clinical paranoia.

Whether these paranoid restricted defenses, which comprise formal paranoid thinking, are themselves in turn the product of underlying repressed trauma is an interesting, but entirely different question.

THE PARANOID COMPANION

To return to Dan. Perhaps because I sensed, intuitively, that his thinking was so restricted, with so few options open, I decided to join him as a companion in his paranoid fantasies. Dan was gratified that I was so willing to carefully examine every detail and every motive of every idea of reference. I suppose it suggested to him that a genuine alliance of paranoid companions had sprung up, that by initiating and seemingly duplicating his paranoid process, I was thereby entering the paranoid system. My hope, of course, was that by so entering and being admitted into Dan's paranoid system I might have a chance of introducing something benign; that by faithfully accompanying him on every paranoid hunt, chasing down every lead with him, but always contriving to steer him to another pathway, I might bring him to the unavoidable conclusion: there is nothing there.

Sometimes it worked, and when it did, Dan was visibly relieved: "I just *loved* that step by step thing you did," he would say.

There are two preconditions which are favorable to this strategy. The first is that your patient genuinely likes and trusts you, that there is an initial strong, positive transference. This is important because the very act of entering another person's paranoid system, means that disturbing material is continually going to be stimulated. To tolerate the logical suspicion that the therapist is interested in such disturbing material primarily as a means of tormenting the patient, strong trust is needed. And in my experience, whenever this strategy had worked, there was an underlying alliance between myself and the patient. Once the strategy had been set up, and a new investigative paranoid alliance had been initiated and accepted by the patient, there was usually a sense of immediate relief that he was no longer alone in his ego-alien world. In itself, this was reassuring: simply the idea of companionship among delusional thoughts was therapeutic. Also, in addition to companionship, the symbiosis implied by the therapist adopting the paranoid style, perhaps served as a transitional step for the patient so far as relinquishing the principal ideas of reference. Perhaps the strategy when it worked, worked in part because it functioned as a *transitional paranoia*. In other words, by accompanying the paranoid step by step, and never deflecting him more than a degree at a time in order to gently steer him toward a less distorted conclusion, there was the compensating security that in spite of partial differences of opinion, much of the paranoid's inner world (Sandler and Rosenblatt 1962; Sandler 1987) was going to be preserved.

The second condition which was favorable to the strategy working, was that your patient be no more ill than what is called borderline psychotic (someone who can move in and out of psychosis) rather than someone entrenched in an encapsulated psychotic paranoia, where the chances of finding the necessary trust to build a paranoid alliance are correspondingly poor. I was therapeutically very lucky, in the case of Dan, that his full-blown psychosis did not occur until two years after we had met and begun to work together. Had it been otherwise, I doubt whether our relationship could have weathered the full two-month storm of his paranoid episode.

A corollary of being able to sustain a therapeutic paranoid collaboration is that there ensues a gradual, subtle change of roles. There is a shift away from the dominating internal threat, the persecuting introject, to a more tolerable analysis of the origins and motives of the alleged persecution. By temporally distancing from the specific persecutory trauma, it moderates the negative affect and allows the patient a second chance to rework, step-by-step, the original paranoid process, but this time assisted by the corrective perspective of the accompanying therapist: for example, in the case of Dan my central interpretation, "Doesn't it seem that Mike would have had to have gone to a great deal of trouble to have gotten Mary to do that? Do you really think you're *that* important to Mike?" It is hoped, by thereby changing roles, that the characteristic noncontextual thinking of the paranoid will be broadened, that it will become increasingly easier for him to reconsider his conclusions about the intentions of his persecutor, than to dwell on the unforgettable pain of being mysteriously tortured.

That was my strategy. As I practiced it, I began to realize how significant were the gaps, the lacunae, in the antecedent process which culminated in the crystallizing paranoid idea; how seriously flawed in his logic and grossly negligent of outstanding contradictory evidence is the paranoid, who presumes to take his scrupulous attention to incriminating detail for granted. By showing him otherwise, it can serve to loosen the rigid shackles of the paranoid process and be thereby therapeutic. You might call this the incidental technique of Cross Examining the Internal Prosecutor in order to shake his testimony (reality hold on the patient); there may even be, as an additional by-product of the technique, a kind of subliminal cognitive matching, which strengthens the therapeutic alliance. Even highly intelligent paranoid patients seem to produce gaping logical flaws (more of the nature of overlooking blatant contradictory evidence which stares them in the face) throughout the entire process, culminating in the consummatory idea of reference.

Each step of the way, deletions of reality and paranoid distortions regularly occur. Because this is sometimes passed over, there is an overemphasis, in the literature, on the idea of reference as being pathognomic of clinical paranoia, and a neglect of the equally pathognomic process preceding the idea of reference. Another way of saying this is that *the paranoid is paranoid long before he arrives at the crystallizing paranoid idea of reference.* Perhaps, it is still more correct to say that paranoia is better defined by the less auspicious preceding process than by the conspicuous distortions which are the end result. That this has been acknowledged, can be seen in the writings of theoreticians such as W.W. Meissner who go so far as to speculate whether the so-called paranoid process

(1978) is actually ubiquitous in psychological development (1987). According to the British psychoanalyst R.D. Laing, one of the prominent characteristics of paranoid ideation is that it involves a failure of feedback. In an early book (1961, p. 178) Laing describes this ingeniously:

> He thinks she thinks that she has managed to trick him into being jealous, but she (1) may not be deceiving him, she might only be pretending to be deceiving him, so (2) he will only pretend to be jealous, but (3) she might be aware that he is aware that she is not sure whether he really is jealous.

In other books, Laing went on to describe what can happen when the failure of feedback in a paranoid interpersonal system, instead of being corrected, begins to spiral (1966, 1970, 1982). In terms of the present discussion, the therapist, by accompanying the paranoid faithfully in his ideation, may be offering what (according to Laing) has been pathologically absent: a corrective feedback. We differ from Laing, who was an admitted disciple of Gregory Bateson (Bateson et al. 1956), in that the corrective feedback is not one of information, but of intimacy.

Intimacy Panic

Is it paradoxical to speak of intimacy and paranoia? Dan showed it was not. Dan showed that the paranoid who dreads intimacy on one level may crave attention on another; and rather than accept indifference may actually prefer the spotlight and the third degree of persecution. Viewed this way, paranoia is a denial of perceived indifference and a defense against the imagined fragmentation that could result from it. Viewed this way, the corrective feedback which the paranoid desperately needs is not the negative attention which he pursues, and provokes, but the intimacy which he dreads and avoids. And in terms of the relationship between therapist and patient, the only corrective intimacy that can be offered, the only positive, more healthy attention which can be given is—empathy.

Robert Stolorow, the self psychologist, has described (Stolorow et al. 1987) the importance of empathy and of continually entering and reentering the empathic field of the patient. Seen in this light, the failure of feedback, pointed to by R.D. Laing, is the failure of empathy, and one reason the technique of becoming a paranoid companion can work is because it adds something that is pathologically absent from the paranoid's field: empathy. Furthermore, it may be that persecutory threat dominates paranoid fantasies *because* of a lack of healthy empathic self-esteem. In other words, paranoia, in yet another defining characteristic, may be seen as a pathological absence of empathy: empathy for oneself and for others.

On the subject of empathy, Otto Kernberg (1987), in his discussion of projection (a central mechanism in paranoia), has alluded to the importance of "lack of empathy with what is projected, and distancing or estrangement from the object as an effective completion of the defensive effort" (p. 94). In terms of our discussion, this lack of empathy and distancing on the part of the projecting paranoid may be what is partially corrected by our introduction of empathy, eventuating in a diminished need for the normal distance normally required in paranoia. If this is so, it may be because the normal defensive distance required by normal or neurotic projection is pathologically intensified by the intimacy panic of the paranoid so that the typical alienation of the other (into the role of a persecuting enemy), can be seen as a guarantee of the defensive need for interpersonal distance. We can now add one more characteristic to our expanding definition of paranoia: when the need for interpersonal distance is so great that it is allowed to become pathological (ego-alien).

Otto Kernberg, on the subject of empathy in paranoid patients, writes (1987, p. 100): "Projective identification, one might say, assures the capacity of empathy under conditions of hatred." Kernberg here is referring to a "primitive" (p. 101) or pathological form of empathy; that is, an empathy which does not relate to the positive aspects of the self, Kohut's (1971) healthy self-esteem, or to the positive aspects of the object.

In our view, a pathological empathy that operates under conditions of hatred and does not relate to the positive aspects of the self nor to the positive aspects of the other, is a contradiction in terms, and is no empathy at all. This can be summarized in the following brief formula, which assumes noncontextual thinking: intimacy panic plus pathological interpersonal distance plus no empathy equals paranoia. The corresponding strategy of joining the paranoid in his fantasies is based on the underlying premise that nothing can be as therapeutic as helping the paranoid to become more empathic to his persecutory objects (both intrapsychic and interpersonal).

Otto Kernberg vividly described an encounter with a hostile paranoid patient who threatened him with violence (1987). As a last resort, Kernberg drew upon a technique he calls confronting the patient with "incompatible realities" (1987, p. 112). This is to point out that the difference in viewpoints between patient and therapist is so wide as to be irreconcilable; that someone (either therapist or patient) must seriously alter his perspective in order for there to be any hope of therapeutically, collaboratively working together again. Kernberg then invites his patient to a joint exploration of where the incompatibility truly lies. We would add it may be helpful to use this technique—not just when the therapist is threatened by a paranoid patient—but specifically when the paranoid patient is threatened by his own persecutory ideas. In other words, to point out that the distance between the paranoid and his object of persecution is so vast as to constitute "incompatible realities"; and that therefore, someone is mad, and that it may be worthwhile to collaboratively search for and to locate where the madness is. This amounts to inviting the paranoid to himself enter the intersubjective field (Stolorow et al. 1987) and to locate, empathically, instead of with his characteristic hatred, the source of the madness.

Again, let's return to Dan and see how all of this is incorporated in what might be called the interpersonal paranoid stance.

The paranoid, who is regularly provocative, threatening, distancing, and rejecting cannot fail to provoke aggression, thereby creating a self-fulfilling prophecy. In this way, paranoia may use an unconscious strategy of guaranteeing distance by alienating the other person. As a corollary of this, the paranoid may select relationships on the basis of their potential for hostility, and may be drawn to people who both promise and maintain a preestablished distance. A lot follows from this. Since hostility guarantees distance, and since paranoid interpersonal relations generally involve mutually reinforcing reciprocal hostility—distance must be guaranteed.

Why distance? One reason appears to be that distance is an important defense against the paranoid's dread of intimacy. It does not matter whether that intimacy is homosexual (as asserted by Freud [1911]) or heterosexual; what is dreaded is the terrifying fantasy of smothering human closeness. As Dan repeatedly showed, the paranoid wants attention, wants to be considered important, wants to be watched, but does not want closeness. What person better fits this description than an enemy or persecutor?

From the standpoint of the double bind, we can say that the central double bind of paranoia is this: the *paranoid is too fragile to be left alone, to be truly autonomous and so needs the comforting illusion of human presence and contact, but is also too fragile to receive, trust, and develop that contact into what is called intimacy.* The internalized persecutor or interpersonal enemy, therefore, can be looked upon as a *pathological resolution* to the double bind of paranoia. Remember, we are always using the idea of the double bind not as the traditional family double bind theorists use it (Bateson et al. 1956)—an unspoken, cognitive clash between conflicting levels of communication—but as a dynamic conflict between incompatible levels of intimacy and relating. In this sense, the double bind of paranoia is a double bind of incompatible levels of intimacy.

In retrospect, much of what transpired with Dan and other paranoid patients I've worked with, fell into place if looked upon as pathological resolutions to the double bind of paranoia. If the paranoid is too fragile to develop an intimate relationship with anyone, but cannot be independently alone, having an enemy can seem a solution. If the paranoid is too fragile to endure more than a fleeting human contact, then relationships which are fixated, frozen, predictable, and offer few surprises, may seem gratifyingly safe. From this angle, the classic persecution of the paranoid may serve a plausible defensive need of stopping the development of any threatening, human intimacy. From this angle, the characteristic, puzzle-solving, murder-mystery, who-dun-it nature of paranoid thinking can be a way of tying a ribbon around a relationship. If the whole point of a relationship (as it often is with paranoids) is simply to determine the guilt and blame, to uncover the hidden, hostile motives of the other—if the relationship is consummated once guilt has been assigned—it is also a beautiful way of denying and excluding the need for intimacy. This can explain why paranoid fantasies often consist of alternating roles of either witness-on-the-stand or prosecutor. Much of paranoid thinking is devoted to the prosecution of the internal prosecutor. While it is often noted in the literature—the degree by which paranoid ideation is divorced from reality and is ego-alien—what is generally underemphasized is how protective and defensive this is for the fear of intimacy.

This defense against intimacy can also be understood in the context of the double bind. Freud speculated (1911) there was one central etiology to paranoia and one defense—the defense of projection against unacceptable homosexual impulses. Yet, if this were the case, there should be a *decline* in paranoid thinking once homosexual impulses were acknowledged and integrated into the personality. Clinical experience, especially in this contemporary age of greater and greater "coming out," often shows the reverse. Self-accepting homosexuals are not necessarily less paranoid than corresponding heterosexuals. They may be more. The real issue may not be denial and projection of repressed homosexual impulses, but both the dread of intimacy and the inability to be alone, that is, the primary double bind of paranoia and the pathological resolution to it, and this may or may not be connected with homosexuality.

Popular culture, in its own way, reflects this view. It is no accident that detective stories and murder mysteries, from the standpoint of serious literature, are notoriously devoid of character development. This may be because the mystery, drama, and suspense of the detective story serve an overlooked but important fictional defensive function: they successfully cover up—by providing so much artificial excitement and stimulation—an underlying pathology and poverty of relating. This, of course, is what we have been saying about paranoid thinking and relating. It is no surprise, therefore, that paranoid thinking resembles nothing so much as a good, old-fashioned detective story. It is another way of saying that detective stories, in terms of pop culture, are fictionalized paranoid adventures. Once you have proven that someone you know (whether in real life or in fiction) is your secret enemy, it is nearly foolproof logic that you must never contemplate intimacy with that person. It can be summed up by saying that while it is characteristic of evolving intimate relationships to be striving to integrate reciprocal closeness, the *reverse* is true of paranoid relating: there is an obsession with the implicit avoidance of intimacy, which is achieved by making the heart and soul of the relationship into a legalistic establishment of the guilt of the enemy.

Carry this one step further and we can understand how some of the underlying anxiety and dread of intimacy driving the paranoid may be transformed into a corresponding anxiety which manifests itself, typically, as the trait of being *fascinated*, almost spellbound with the puzzlelike character of their relationships (as they see them). By trying so hard to figure out the clues and solve the detective storylike mystery of their relationships, the paranoid may also be unconsciously striving to drain off and perhaps exhaust an uncontrollable anxiety in the face of almost any human contact.

In turn, this may explain why the paranoid's account of his relationships and, especially, of his fantasies resembles nothing so much as *plot outlines*. Missing are the multidimensions, richness, and fullness which are basic to and define most human relationships. Moreover, the plots are rigidly circumscribed and rigorously edited, with few allowable variations.

Years ago, when I was a student attending several therapy institutes in New York City, I took a seminar in projective testing. The teacher, a well-known expert in projective testing, held up before the class a drawing of a tree (in the House-Tree-Person test) executed by a clinically diagnosed paranoid man. The roots of the depicted tree appeared to be like powerful talons crawling across the surface of the ground. Those of us who got the message gave a small collective shudder. All the teacher said was, "notice the roots lie on the *outside* of the ground."

It was a telling point which stayed with me. So much of paranoid thinking and relating have this quality of being outside, not making contact; lying beyond the pale of what is considered human. It is not unfair to say that paranoid thinking displays an intrinsically alien, almost Martian quality, and these ego-alien characteristics may not be exclusively the end results of prior cognitive or structural weakness. Perhaps, they are defenses, however maladaptive. Perhaps their function is to create a basically grotesque, inhuman parody of intimacy which is not so much ego-alien, as *inhuman*. If this is so, the comic book, Martian, murder-mystery quality so often observed in the paranoid style, may not be only the end result of a psychical breakdown, but a necessary defensive artifice as well to preserve a powerful, dramatically alive, but essentially nonintimate relationship. It is a remarkable fact that many of the classic signs in projective testing which are diagnostic of clinical paranoia—invisible watching eyes, lofty aerial perspective, a pervasive sense of partially hidden, evil secrecy—are all descriptive of *nonhuman* relationships. It is not nearly enough to say they are ego-alien. It is more accurate to say that listening to a paranoid patient is like listening to someone describe a relationship that one is having with an almost nonhuman alien.

Consider this: what is less personal, less human, less intimate than a relationship with someone who seems to be trying to poison, torture, or murder you? But what is more dramatic? In this sense, paranoid ideation may be viewed as a diabolical creation, a kind of evil little story about what one person is doing to another. The artist, like Dan, simply raises this to a higher level, but the mechanism is the same. The mechanism, however, is not restricted to paranoid pathology. Our present-day adult love affair with action–murder–violence cinema, which can be traced back to a childhood fascination with the cruelty of fairy tales and, later, comic books, may also point to a more normal usage of a similar paranoid mechanism; that is, to try to feel alive, when one is too frightened or too tired to be otherwise humanly intimate, by engaging in a vicarious paranoid entertainment. By vicarious paranoid entertainment, we refer to the current vogue of action–murder–violence cinema. Just as Freud sometimes spoke of a civilization's collective neurosis (1928), our widespread obsession with pop culture scenarios of violence may be a media-sanctioned, collective paranoia.

Underlying the intimacy panic of paranoia and the dread of contact is what can only be called a pathological mistrust. So much attention has been focused on the cognitive distortions of paranoid ideas of reference or the underlying pathology of primitive projection, that it is sometimes overlooked how powerful an ingredient is the paranoid's mistrust; and how far-reaching are its ramifications. If you are saying, as the paranoid does, that someone is trying to murder, poison, or control your brain, you are also saying, in however a baroque, soap-operaish way, that you could not conceivably trust someone less. What is the ultimate betrayal of one person by another if not murder? What is the antithesis of nurturing intimacy if not sadism, torture, and perpetrated humiliation? And if these are the frequent fantasies of paranoids, what are they about if not dramatizations of the extreme danger someone is in if involved with a supremely and diabolically untrustworthy person? It is a theme the movies never tire of portraying. *The Godfather, Taxi Driver, Raging Bull,* instead of depicting supposedly sociologically interesting criminal subcultures, are really about something so banal and fundamental as mistrust: yet something so unnervingly widespread in contemporary society that unless dressed up in layer after layer of macabre paranoid plot, it would really scare people away.

For all of these reasons, as a therapist, you often experience the paranoid patient as the dramatist and yourself as the audience. You find yourself waiting for the next scene, the next torturer, the next conspiratorial plot twist to develop. The biggest confirming clue of all which the paranoid is waiting for is the confirmation that his therapist believes him. If the paranoid's transference is that he perpetually is on the witness stand, then the therapist's complementary countertransference often is that he is becoming what he can not become—a *jury*.

When the paranoid enters into a full-blown episode, as Dan did for two months, therapy finds itself, whether it wants to or not, in the crisis mode. There is then extraordinary pressure on the therapist to be on the side of the patient, to rescue him; to prove that one has not defected to the enemy camp. It is a dilemma for the therapist that what the patient means by loyalty is that the therapist emotionally accept the specific paranoid ideas and become a partisan. Even if the therapist manages not to become a partisan and not to thereby offend the patient, he is forced to deal in constant crisis intervention. If someone feels as though he is hanging from a cliff edge, then only one frame of reference in therapy is possible: Does what is happening or being said by the therapist help me to hang on or does it allow me to fall off? In such an endangered atmosphere insight, which is always threatening to the paranoid, can become so irrelevant as to appear not only useless but even intrusive. It then becomes itself grist for the paranoia: "Why is he analyzing me instead of helping me?"

In such an endangered atmosphere, transference to the therapist can become nearly psychotic as the paranoid looks to therapy as a literal last resort and lifesaver before being killed, tortured, or carted off to the hospital. At this point, therapy ends with the paranoid. They either leave, are referred to a psychiatrist, or actually do wind up in the hands of the police or in a hospital. The fact none of these things happened with Dan, as I've already said, must be attributed to the preceding two years during which we had worked intensively together and as closely as we could.

I had never seen Dan so happy, relieved, and connected to me as when he finally came out of his full-blown episode. Yet, it is a sad measure of the paranoid's dread of intimacy, that he can feel most interpersonally alive only when he is in the process of being rescued from the brink of annihilation.

4
The Death of an Artist

Harry's Denial

Nothing is as painful as to sit, certain that there is nothing you can do about it, and watch your patient die. After all, therapy is based on trust, trust is based on hope, but where can that be found in the radical existential condition of knowing you are terminally ill? It is therefore hard, as a therapist, not to feel useless, pointless, sometimes absurdly irrelevant; to even wonder just who is the patient here and whether it is you who really needs someone to help get him through an unmanageable, unbearable experience.

    I had little idea that this is what I would be getting into when I first met Harry, and from the looks of Harry—his thoughtful, mannered, but comical air of sardonically dismissing everything, light or serious, that came his way with the best collegiate humor he could muster—neither did he. Far from being in good spirits, he was downright depressed. The depression, though, seemed boyish and petulant: in his presence you never felt the downward pull, the drag and gravity of the truly and chronically hopeless. Accordingly, I assumed upon meeting Harry that I was meeting just another young man, troubled to be sure as all patients were, but someone with a typically imprecise but undeniable future.

And Harry did nothing to dissuade this. Six months earlier, prior to our first session, he had alarmingly begun coughing up significant quantities of blood, and rushed himself to the hospital. X-rays revealed a suspicious spot on his right lung. A biopsy revealed a malignancy. The operation that was immediately ordered removed a major portion of his right lung but the surgeon who performed it pronounced it an unqualified success. Harry had no reason to worry about the recurrence of cancer; he had been the lucky recipient of what was called a surgical cure. And if that weren't enough, there was the indisputable fact that everyone in his family had "constitutions like horses."

No, Harry wasn't worried about his future from the standpoint of longevity. He was going to be around for a long time. What did worry him, though, was not his current depression—that he could handle—but the possibility it could grow into something seriously debilitating. Harry could remember two such episodes, each lasting for a period of months: the first when he was twenty years old and the last, three years ago, when he was twenty-five. Both times he felt more than numb (his present feeling) he felt paralyzed, psychologically dead. It was all he could do to crawl out of bed in the morning and function on the lowest possible survival level. If he could do that, he felt good about himself because he prided himself on being a durable, tenacious loner, someone who could take care of himself under any circumstances. It followed that Harry, in the grip of his initial major depression, resisted outside help, and that, although only twenty, he was confident he could administer an adequate self-cure. Only when vigorous efforts along these lines—relaxation exercises, intense physical activity, stepped-up socializing, a new diet—consecutively failed did he finally turn to psychotherapy and then psychiatry.

At the age of twenty, Harry appraised psychotherapy to have

THE DEATH OF AN ARTIST

been an enjoyable intellectual exchange but one that did little for his depression. He respected psychiatrists even less, but he believed that one of the antidepressants which were prescribed did in fact help to alleviate his depression.

I asked Harry the name of the antidepressant which had been helpful and saw my question waved aside. That's not why he had come to see me. He had already made contact with a psychiatrist in New York, and any time he wanted to, he could have his prescription for an antidepressant refilled. What he wanted from me was something different: he wanted to trace back the roots of his depression, psychologically, to his early childhood relationship with his mother which he felt certain contained the key, in order to better understand, control, and (hopefully) nip in the bud the onset of any subsequent, major depression.

Was I such a man, the man he was looking for? In our first session, in the space of just thirty minutes of knowing me, Harry felt comfortable enough to present his first intellectual challenge. More would follow. Turning therapy into a cerebral contest was a distinct pleasure for Harry and a game at which he excelled. Many months later, when he was truly sick, when our relationship had been necessarily, strategically reduced to an urgent collaboration to prolong his survival—he would continue to savor those moments when my sense of loss at what to say or how to help struck him as both ironically amusing and faintly endearing. "Poor Jerry," he would comment, acting for all the world like a patient, long-suffering, but consoling parent.

Since neither Harry nor I knew how sick he was, how sick he was about to become, I was content to listen to his story, not realizing how short the time of his narrative would be.

Harry began at the beginning. He was born in New Jersey. His mother was a housewife, a fiercely intelligent woman who was determined to improve her station. His father, whom Harry hardly remembers, was an unambitious bookkeeper who relocated to Miami when his company did. There was a brother, four years older, destined to be a biofeedback psychologist, whom Harry believed discovered his future career in the midst of enthusiastically modifying his younger brother's behavior. One year after the family moved to Miami, when Harry was four, his father died of cancer. He has vague memories of there being a family crisis, if not an emotional at least a financial crisis. Later, he would understand that for a number of years it had been necessary to supplement the family income with a welfare subsidy. But for the present, it only meant that he suddenly found himself eating far more peanut butter sandwiches than he could possibly want, becoming acutely aware for the first time that his brother, who was already proficient at anticipating and reasonably providing whatever Harry needed, was nevertheless a bully and, occasionally, a sadistic disciplinarian.

The biggest disappointment of all occurred when his mother decided to return to college and complete the undergraduate studies she had interrupted when she got married. To eight-year-old Harry, such behavior could only be interpreted as child abandonment and not the meritorious self-improvement his mother solemnly insisted upon; and by this time he knew he was excessively attached to his mother, as well as being the apple of her eye. So he would bide his time, manufacture things to do, which was easy because he had so many intellectual interests, stay as far away as he could from the clutches of his brother's intrusive helpfulness, and wait until his mother came home first from school and then her job.

When she did arrive, there would be plenty of time. She loved closeting herself with her young son, whom she regarded as precociously intelligent, and trying to devise new and better ways of cultivating his development which already was ahead of schedule. Harry didn't mind performing for his mother. He could read fluently by the time he was five, so it was relatively simple for him to handle the intellectual challenges his mother regularly posed for him: to learn the capitals of each of the states of the United States, to memorize the overall geography of the world, to master the principal dates in history, to read the great novels of world literature and compose brief, coherent book reports, and even tackle advanced mathematics several years beyond his present grade level. None of it was really difficult for Harry. In retrospect, it seemed he had effortlessly ascended, almost by natural right, to the throne of being the family intellectual.

Much more important to Harry was the second privileged position he had come to occupy with his mother, mainly because it was the one he had to work so hard and so dearly to achieve: that of being her most trusted, emotional confidante. From around the age of twelve on, the rest of Harry's personality caught up with his overtrained intelligence. He was not only bright, he was also extremely creative, sensitive, imaginative, and artistic. Harry could not only read books, he could read people. The most precious knowledge of all was his understanding, finally, of his mother with a kind of depth that again outmatched his years. It dawned on Harry how lonely and bitter was his mother, how, underlying her embattled determination to raise the cultural standards of herself and her children, was her own uneasy perception of just how insecure, anxious, and fragile she was. Harry now saw that his mother's need for him was more than a selfless need to elevate her son; it was a need to sustain herself, to keep herself afloat by holding onto her son as though he were a lifesaver.

Harry had a new role now, one that far outshone being the family intellectual. He would shelve his own worries and feelings—he could manage those—and devote himself to helping his mother get through her life.

Years later, he would realize how much of himself he had lost in the process of saving his mother, but for the time being he was exhilarated to be of such precocious service. Yet, if he was a linchpin at home, he was something else; he was an odd man out at school. Harry went to a very tough school in a very poor section of Miami where survival in the street, and not education, was the priority. As Harry would put it to me, "They just didn't get me." Of medium height and very slight build when I met him, he was a good five inches shorter as a teenager and felt childish compared with his much more physically mature classmates. Compounding the mismatch, Harry could not discover a single interest he held in common with his peers. He played chess, liked to solve puzzles of all kinds, devoured whatever book he happened to lay his hands on, and was already experimenting with what would be his artistic calling—playwrighting. He detested sports which he found incomprehensible. He wouldn't physically fight, even if he had to, and even if he could. It wasn't that he was afraid, it was that he was so removed, so detached from the world of violent, physical action that he could not conceive of himself doing it. And listening to Harry as he told me this in the session, I did not hesitate to believe him. He had a quality I have rarely seen that I can only call abstract fearlessness; that is, once he made up his mind to do something, and this was borne out on a number of occasions during the time I knew him, he would do almost anything.

Because of all of this, Harry's classmates did not know what to make of him, nor what to do with him. He was different, he was weird, maybe he was gay, but he wasn't different in an interesting way and he certainly wasn't one of them. He wasn't even interesting enough (because he was too small) to be picked on or bullied, so they collectively shunned him, quietly sneering as he passed by in the corridor.

Harry believed one incident, in particular, turned things around for him, and during the session in which he described it, occurring several months after I had met him, he was more animated than I had ever seen him. Harry had decided, against the protests of two friends whom he dragged along, to attend a weekend dance sponsored by his high school, but in a section of town where few white people went. He recognized it was an act of some daring, but he convinced himself and his friends there had to be some white people on the huge gymnasium dance floor, and, besides, he would be recognized if not welcomed by his classmates, many of whom undoubtedly would be there.

No one (except Harry) guessed the real reason: he loved to dance, wildly and creatively, mostly in the privacy of his bedroom, and to dance with a black girl was a favorite and powerful erotic fantasy. Now, at the age of sixteen, it was going to come true. Understandably, Harry was nervous, not terrified as were his two friends, as he carefully made his way along the margin of the populated dance floor. Among hundreds of mostly teenagers, Harry did not see another white face. He saw plenty of classmates, who either glared at him or snickered, but no one he could identify as a friend and certainly no one who seemed happy he was there. His two friends were urging him, really pestering him, to get out of there while they could, but Harry waited, not knowing what he was going to do, but knowing he had to do something.

He didn't have to wait long. A black girl, tough and several inches taller than Harry, who at least acknowledged his existence in the school corridors in a rough bantering way, came up to him. Was he here to watch, or to dance? "Dance," said Harry, already feeling flustered but excited, knowing, as he trailed behind her, he had not been invited to dance, he had been invited to a challenge. In a corner of the dance floor, the black girl (assuming the lead) executed what she considered a complicated, show-offy step and then stopped, as though daring her partner to keep pace with her. Almost instantaneously Harry copied her step and then improvised a flourish of his own. Surprised, a bit angry, and now seriously competitive, she threw herself into a whirling, chaotic series of steps that left her breathless at the finish. Yet, even before she had finished, almost perfectly mirroring the spirit of her styleless, crazed dance, Harry had picked up her tempo and used it to launch into his own weird, wonderfully creative, private choreography. At its conclusion, the black girl, who recognized she was being completely outshone, in spite of herself, laughed appreciatively.

By now, a curious crowd, which continued to grow, had formed a circle around Harry whom they no longer could simply categorize. He was a white boy, but he didn't dance like one. He didn't dance like a black boy either. He danced like no one they had ever seen, and what's more, his dancing excited them. They would test him out. Over the next half hour, one after the other, about ten black girls in all challenged him in what Harry proudly remembered as a "dance-off." Not only did he emerge unscathed and undefeated, but he had given birth to a reputation and inspired a loyalty, especially among the black girls who had danced with him, that would follow him and cushion his way through his remaining year and a half in high school.

The "dance-off" was perhaps the most exhilarating experience and memory brought forth into therapy up until that point. By now, after several months, Harry had settled comfortably into his self-appointed role: he was part raconteur, part educator as he leisurely attempted to trace back the roots of his current depression to his early childhood. It was true I was a professional, a therapist, but more important (to Harry), I was a colleague, someone he had hired to accompany him on an intellectual, archaeological expedition as we sifted through the meaningful relics of his past. He didn't mind; in fact he enjoyed alternating, sprinkling this historical account with lively reflections on his contemporary state of being. In particular, he would dwell on the banality of his life as he saw it; the great difficulty he experienced in motivating himself to do anything; and the excruciating, laborious process he was forced to endure before he could make even the tiniest of decisions.

Harry also talked about his mind, as few patients do, as though it were an independently existing domain with a life force of its own. He spoke of the books he adored. Especially intriguing to him were vampire novels, in vogue at that time, and there was one entire session which he devoted to a scholarly rumination on the vicissitudes of vampire lore. When he was finished, I pointed out that perhaps, in addition, his relish for the subject was flavored by a personal investment: that he had often spoken of sections of his body and mind as being frozen with depression; that he had recently survived a brush with death, when a large, cancerous mass from his right lung was surgically removed; and that, therefore, since vampires are archetypal symbols of being dead yet alive, perhaps they represented to him an appealing denial and antidote for both the recurrence of cancer and the onset of another major depression.

A light seemed to go off in Harry's head. He gave me a long look, followed by a slow nod. Whenever an interpretation seemed to him to be pleasingly on target, he had a way of making known to me the precise degree of his appreciation; as though he had his private four-star rating system in reserve to fairly but critically be applied whenever I was bold enough to hazard an interpretation on a subject he considered himself to be the world's greatest expert in: his mind. And I was sufficiently in touch with my own countertransference to realize that whenever Harry—who was, undoubtedly, quirks and all, one of my favorite patients—responded with a four-star nod following one of my interpretations, I was much too gratified.

Nevertheless, for those first few months, therapy (according to Harry and myself) was proceeding at a generally satisfying pace and I was content to follow him wherever he went. He was twenty-eight years old and looked in fine health. Neither of us knew that precious time was ticking away. Letting Harry, in his leisurely ironic fashion, continue his story seemed the thing to do.

The notoriety he had won for his performance at the "dance-off" made life in the blackboard jungle considerably less hazardous, and by the time he graduated from high school he felt confident he could survive in the outside world as well. He postponed matriculating at Columbia University, where he had not only been accepted but accorded a full scholarship, and decided to experience life instead. He still considered himself his mother's most reliable protector, but he could no longer function under the symbiotic umbrella of a mother–son relationship, he had to stake out his own loner's existence, and he preferred to do it as far away as possible. At the age of seventeen he officially left home and proceeded to hitchhike to New York City. He spent two months on the road. The life-style he was adopting—what Harry would later refer to as his first major existential decision—was that of "intellectual hobo." When he finally arrived in New York City, he was penniless and without resources, but the thought of asking his mother for subsidization, seeming like spineless surrender, was unthinkable. In short order, he became, instead, a connoisseur of meaningless and often humiliating odd jobs: working, variously, as a busboy, dishwasher, waiter, tour guide, usher, self-employed house cleaner, and telemarketer. The tougher the job and the higher the turnover, the more Harry prided himself on his loner's ability to survive.

He did not lack friends, either. His unrelenting, humorously snobbish satirization of just about everything New Yorkish, endeared him to the artistic crowd he was running with and made his passage from resident family intellectual to witty social iconoclast a swift one. He was getting a new kind of attention and a new kind of notoriety. When he completed his first full-length play at the age of twenty and immediately had it produced in an Off-Off Broadway loft, everyone was amazed except Harry, who had come to believe more and more, that life was going to be lived on his terms.

He had the survivor's instincts, the willpower, and especially the intelligence to carry it through. He would cash in on the full scholarship he had been awarded by Columbia University but he would matriculate at his own pace. Accordingly, about once every year or two he would devise a plausible leave of absence story acceptable to the university faculty and use it to return full time to his diverse, extracurricular pursuits. It accounted for the fact that Harry, admittedly a brilliant student, at the age of twenty-eight, after nearly a decade of matriculation at Columbia University, was still six months shy of necessary graduation credits.

When months had passed, and I had yet to hear of a single sexual adventure, I decided—banking on the fact he was anything but shy—to ask about it. Harry smiled, pleased with my interest, welcoming the opportunity to reveal another of his odd-ball, decadent tastes. Yes, he liked women, but women considerably older than he was—as much as twenty-five to thirty-five years older. He didn't know why, didn't know whether it was some mother–son attraction, but knew he wasn't interested in having it reduced to some Freudian paradigm.

And the reason he hadn't, up until now, spoken of sexual activity was quite simple: he had been celibate for the past six months. The woman he was presently seeing—Harry was careful not to call her his girl friend—was a retired attorney. She was sixty-one years old. Harry had met her about a year ago at one of the all-ages-welcome dance/disco social gatherings he regularly attended. On his first date, his unerring instinct in such matters told him to bring her a rose. Three days later she invited him to have intercourse with her, something she had not permitted herself to do for the last fifteen years. Two weeks later, when she realized that not only would he not marry her but that he had scant emotional interest in her, she became sadly resigned that, in order to keep him, she would have to principally attend to his needs. As compensation, Harry spent time with her, and once a month slept with her.

The depression that brought him back to therapy had set in about six months ago. He became so sexually turned off that it became impossible to have intercourse with her. It was all he could do to occasionally lie in bed with her, put his arms around her, or fondle her breasts.

Four months had now passed since Harry had started therapy. He was beginning to see connections between his early family history, his feelings of depression, his relationship with himself, his relationship with older women. We both, as I've mentioned, thought there would be time enough to develop any and all such connections. But when he got sick, he got sick fast.

Although he had come into therapy following a relatively recent lung operation, there had never been the slightest hint of bronchial distress. So it was only a mild surprise, and no threat at all, when Harry—about five minutes before a session was scheduled to end—began to cough. It sounded like any other cough. Harry motioned for me to start talking, to take over so as not to waste any valuable time on something so trivially interfering as a cough. I began to say something. When the cough not only did not abate, but steadily worsened I offered to bring him a glass of water. He shook his head no, and himself disappeared in the bathroom for several minutes. Through the door I heard the cough continue uninterrupted, and when Harry emerged, still coughing, he pointed ineffectually to the clock on the bookcase. I understood immediately that he was alluding to the fact there was still time left in the session, but that he would be unable to benefit by it as he was no longer able to speak. Since he was a stickler for punctuality and ceremony and would not leave, no matter how incapacitated, without authoritative permission, I ventured it might be better if we terminated the session a few minutes earlier than usual. Harry immediately nodded agreement, sprang from the couch, and by now coughing furiously, left the office.

When Harry not only failed to keep his next scheduled appointment three days later, but did not even leave a message—something he had never done—I realized something was radically wrong. I left my own message on his answering machine, urging him to contact me. When there was no response, when he missed his second consecutive appointment, I tried the telemarketing firm which Harry had told me he periodically moonlighted for. Yes, he was presently working there part-time. No, he was unavailable, in fact, he had been unexplainably missing from work for over a week.

I had two weeks to ponder the mystery, before Harry finally did telephone me. He had been in St. Vincent's Hospital for a week, perhaps more, he couldn't be sure, he was still on drugs. Harry spoke clearly, but laboriously. He realized he should have contacted me, but he was sorry, he could not. After he had left me, following his coughing fit in my office, he had gone directly home where he had ample medicinal supplies. He did not think he would have difficulty treating something so simple as a bad cough. Two days later, when his coughing had turned into bouts of vomiting, when his temperature had climbed to 104 degrees, when he experienced the worst panic attack of his life, when he developed a tremor in his hands, even Harry, the incorrigible loner, was scared.

He was certain there could not be any connection between what was presently the matter with him and his recent lung cancer but he had to see a doctor (and he had no one else), so he contacted the surgeon who had operated on him, who immediately ordered extensive tests. One of the tests was a CAT scan which revealed an unexpectedly large tumor lodged so deep in the brain that it was inoperable. "They can't be sure it's cancerous." He sounded sleepy but defiant. He started to lecture me on the kinds of nonmalignant brain tumors (obviously he had already done considerable research on the subject), but felt too exhausted to continue. He would talk to me in full when he got out of the hospital. In the interim, I was welcome to contact his surgeon who would fill me in on his medical progress.

As soon as I got off the telephone with Harry, I dialed the number he had given me for his surgeon. For the first time, I had the uneasy feeling that I could no longer trust Harry to be even a mildly objective reporter when it came to the state of his health. The surgeon who came on the line did nothing to alleviate my anxiety. He sounded young, ambitious, officious, impersonal, and in a very big hurry. What information he gave was rattled off, and he made it clear he had no interest in discussing anything. Yes, the tumor was inoperable. No, it didn't matter. It was cancerous, he was certain. Harry was dying, and soon. When I wanted to know if Harry knew as much, that is, if he had told him, the surgeon did not bother to hide his irritation. "Yes, I did. Look, he has encephalitis. He's undergoing a personality change. He doesn't remember things. He's clinically depressed."

Although I wasn't sure if Harry's doctor was more interested in saving his reputation than in saving his patient, the telephone conversation had taught me one invaluable thing: Harry was into far greater denial than I had ever known him to be. I wanted, on the one hand, very much to meet with him again, so as to help him with this, if I could; on the other hand, felt it was even more important that I respect his sickness, his wish to be left alone until ready, on his own terms, to see me.

So I waited, not entirely sure that my patient was even alive. After about two weeks, I received a second telephone call, not from Harry, but from Harry's psychiatrist, the one he told me he had contacted for an antidepressant prescription prior to first seeing me. By yet another coincidence (showing how small the world of mental health professionals, even in a city the size of New York, can be) I happened to know this man. Eight years earlier, I had participated in a seminar on psychopharmacology for the lay therapist led by this very psychiatrist. At the time, I found him to be a rare combination of scholar-practitioner: someone who had at his fingertips a wealth of up-to-date knowledge on the latest psychotropic medications, as well as an old-fashioned, family physician's dedication to work steadfastly in the best interests of his patient.

Now, eight years later, I found his integrity intact. He spent well over an hour on the telephone with me (when you are lucky if a consulting physician—as witness Harry's surgeon—gives you a good five free minutes). Harry had asked him to call me. He had been in contact with him for nearly a month (I then realized Harry had withheld telling me this, perhaps fearing it would be perceived as a breach of loyalty).

In detail, and with genuine concern, the psychiatrist recounted how he had endeavored to treat Harry for his unexplainable anxiety attack following his coughing fit in my office. Although he had prescribed several reliably effective antianxiety medications, he frankly admitted he had never seen anyone in his experience (and it was vast) as intractable as Harry. He speculated that the anxiety might be purely neurological, a by-product of the encephalitis. He acknowledged, sadly, that Harry would undoubtedly soon die as the cancerous tumor metastasized in his brain. However, before that time, he might become progressively, totally incapacitated, depending on how rapidly and extensively his brain functions were damaged. Therefore, it was advisable he have some family member—in this case, his mother, who had recently relocated to Philadelphia—nearby who could take care of Harry should he become unable to do so himself.

As a matter of fact, the psychiatrist had already had another long talk (at Harry's request) with his mother just the other night. It had been decided by all parties concerned that Harry would first move in almost immediately with his mother in Philadelphia, and thereupon check in with a local hospital for additional tests and close monitoring. The local hospital was reputed to possess an excellent cancer wing, which could provide whatever care would be deemed necessary.

It took a while, but it gradually registered on me that without the courtesy of a prior consultation, my patient had been preempted by the psychiatrist: a kind, conscientious man to be sure, but someone who shared the prevailing prejudice of the majority of psychiatrists that psychotherapy at best is and should be the handmaiden of biological psychiatry—and that, of course, meant essentially, the prescription and monitoring of the preferred medication. Before letting my patient go, therefore, I had to assert the benefits, as I saw them, which Harry had derived from psychotherapy, and I stated my conviction that he continue his therapy in Philadelphia. "He can always do that," the psychiatrist said, softly, yet firmly, "but right now, medical treatment is what he needs."

Two days later Harry called to say goodbye. He was off to Philadelphia; given the circumstances it was the best thing, but he wanted to thank me for all I had done. Agreeing that it sounded like a good idea, I encouraged him to continue his therapy in Philadelphia whenever he felt up to it, and invited him to keep in contact by telephone should he ever feel the need to speak to me.

I was certain when I hung up I would never see Harry again, and that probably I would always be somewhat in the dark as to whether he had died or was somehow hanging on to life. It is an understatement to say I was surprised when Harry called me up ten days later to resume therapy. He was back in New York and living in his old apartment. He was back in Columbia, determined, if he could, to at long last complete his undergraduate studies. He was even back at his evening part-time telemarketing job, at least for the present, for as long as he could stand it.

When You Know You're About to Die

It had been over a month since Harry had been seized in my office by a spasm of unstoppable coughing. I could see the difference. He was at least ten, maybe thirteen, pounds lighter. Since he was quite thin to begin with, he looked—if not cadaverous—distressingly gaunt. Although as clear-headed and precise in speech as ever, he was now noticeably, almost deliberately sluggish, as though even the tiniest movement might prove expensive and therefore had to be calculated in advance. In part, the sluggishness could be attributed to the fact he was being heavily medicated: he was taking drugs, prescribed by his psychiatrist, for his continuing and abnormally high level of anxiety, and he was taking drugs, prescribed by his surgeon, to inhibit the growth of the tumor in his brain.

In spite of which, he was perfectly articulate as he retold the brief, bewildering odyssey of the past ten days. He had gone, as he said he would, to Philadelphia and moved in with his mother, who was doing her best to curtail her palpable hysteria that she was on the brink of losing her precious son. The bed that was supposed to be waiting for him in the cancer ward of the local hospital had been mistakenly assigned to someone else, and Harry was told that it would be weeks, perhaps longer, before another one could be allocated. Harry took it as long as he could (which was roughly seven days)—the idea that he had chosen to live as a ward in the shadow of his mother's care, someone who had forfeited his natural right to make his own life and death decisions.

Then, thanking his mother as diplomatically as he could for all she had tried to do, he returned to his own home in New York. He would function, he had decided, autonomously, until no longer able to do so. So he recontacted his startled psychiatrist, who immediately upped the dosage of his antianxiety medication, and reestablished a schedule of regular visits with his surgeon to monitor the growth of the tumor in his brain. Whatever laboratory tests were needed could be done far more quickly and efficiently in New York than Philadelphia, and should he need rehospitalization, he was certain a bed (through his surgeon) would be made available.

In defiance of the tumor lodged in his brain, Harry was insisting on being his old self. He was taking charge of his own treatment plan, he was critically appraising every move of his doctors, and he was conducting his own independent research into the etiology and possible management of brain tumors. Over and over again, he stressed that the tumor was inoperable, that they could only speculate but could not be certain it was cancerous, and that therefore he had no choice but to conduct his life as though he were going to live and not die. As his therapist, I was therefore faced with the dilemma of whether to confront his defense mechanism of denial, and perhaps undermine something vital to his resolve to carry on, or tacitly collude in the illusion that he was not dying and thereby use therapy to manipulate an indispensable truth.

It was a dilemma I did not find difficult to unravel. Until that time when Harry seemed ready to face the fact of his death, I would plant seeds designed to open and fertilize his mind to at least the possibility he might be denying a very unwanted fate. For example, whenever Harry would lecture me on the variety of benign brain tumors (which he did frequently and with expert obsessiveness) I would occasionally ask him, "What does your doctor say about the tumor in your brain—does he think it's benign or malignant?" It never failed to surprise me that so well-defended was Harry that he could respond to my portentous question with seemingly unruffled dismissiveness: "You know doctors, they're notoriously conservative. He probably says it's cancer in order to cover himself in case he says it isn't but he turns out to be mistaken."

The Good Soldier

I saw Harry for about six more months. From what I could gather, his condition somewhat stabilized. He did not go into remission (as Harry stubbornly insisted) and he was steadily deteriorating (according to his doctors), but the deterioration must have been slight because I could hardly notice it, and I was constantly watching for it. Except for the occasional lapse, when he would call up an hour or two before the session to state he was too weak to get out of bed and therefore would have to cancel, he came regularly to therapy. He came as regularly as healthy patients with healthy, nontumorous brains. Of course, he had to pay a price for such constancy: it took him an exorbitantly long time to get from his door to my door, and when it came to climbing the three flights of stairs leading to my office, he would sometimes allocate as much as five minutes to accomplish it.

What struck me was the unwavering single-mindedness with which Harry seemed to be carrying out his soldierly resolve to live his life as independently as he could right up until the end, whenever that would be. During the final six months that I saw him, Harry spoke about the same things in therapy he had always spoken about. Except now, everything had a little existential frame around it.

Of course, he continued to deny that he was dying, but over the months his resistance noticeably softened. More and more he chose to speculate on dying, becoming fascinated with what the actual experiential moment of dying would be like. He went so far as to present me with a theory: the actual moment of dying, because it would constitute such an unprecedented total release from all existing tensions, would therefore be experientially pleasurable to a magnificent degree. Although I had to wonder if this was more of Harry's denial of death, I found myself touched by his ability to poetically philosophize, to take time off so to speak from the gravest of illnesses.

During this final period, Harry's relationship to me became closer. He was more open, more vulnerable, as well as more angry and more demanding. At times, when he looked as though he had fallen into a bottomless well of hopelessness, he would fix me with a terrible, unspoken, ice-cold stare. It was as though he were saying, "You're my therapist. So, what are you going to do?" Those were the times that were most painful for me, when for all the world I could not think of what possible benefit therapy or myself could offer a man whose brain was in the process of being eaten up by cancer. Fortunately, for me, Harry was too kind to let the moment last and he would get me off the hook by letting go of his anger.

That was one side of the coin. The other was surprising tenderness on the part of Harry, and, sometimes, even poignancy. One such occasion, I remember in particular. It occurred about a month prior to the last time I saw him. He had just received the results of some extensive laboratory tests, including some critical blood workup. The results could not have been more demoralizing. The cancer, it seemed, was metastasizing not only in his brain, but in his body. After reflecting upon this for a few moments, with only a trace of wistful regret, Harry said, "You know, I'm sick. I'm really sick." That was the closest, in the year I knew him, that he came to acknowledging that he was truly about to die.

There are two incidents, among many, that in retrospect, and from as objective a clinical stance as I can muster, I regard as genuinely remarkable. The first such incident occurred approximately one month after Harry had returned from Philadelphia and resumed therapy with me. Good soldier though he undoubtedly was, he reluctantly was forced to concede he could not realistically maintain his former schedule. Some losses would have to be cut. He began by officially terminating his symbiotic mother–son relationship with his sixty-one-year-old platonic companion. It was refreshingly simple, and gratifyingly, mutually beneficial. Next, he quit his part-time evening job as a telemarketing supervisor. Harry had often caricaturized the upsurge of such telemarketing firms as contemporary "neosweatshops."

The free time thereby created enabled him to join one of the various cancer self-help groups now available in New York City. It was there that he got to know Susan, a twenty-five-year-old graduate student who was highly susceptible to periodic skin cancers. Harry joked that this was the first woman younger than himself whom he had dated in the past ten years. Although she was in complete remission, and her prognosis was one of the most promising for cancer patients, she did not hesitate to begin an apparently serious relationship with Harry, knowing full well he was terminally ill (even if he didn't).

What amazed me, was not that he could achieve a relationship while dying, but that he could achieve a quantum jump in the level of his intimacy. For this relationship, from everything that he told me (and he discussed it at length in therapy), was immeasurably closer to authentic, reciprocal love than anything he had come close to experiencing; and despite the fact it was an obvious, romantic long shot with considerable odds against it, it endured as long as Harry did. Which, in turn, would prompt me to deliver my favorite, central interpretation which often would elicit in him (as in me) a manifest sense of genuine meaningful contentment: "You know, you've never been so healthy (psychologically) or functioned so well as since you received your diagnosis of a tumor in the brain."

The second remarkable incident occurred a few weeks before the last time I ever saw him. After ten years of matriculation, Harry had at long last graduated from Columbia. Not only that, he had just been awarded a Phi Beta Kappa key. He was more pleased and proud than I had ever seen him. I could not help sharing and rejoicing a little bit in this with him. I knew he was more than bright, he was brilliant, but that he could continue to maintain the academic standards necessary to achieve a Phi Beta Kappa key while carrying a cancerous tumor in his brain seemed incredible to me.

But there was more to tell. Harry had accepted an invitation to address a group of college students on the subject of dealing with and facing up to serious illness. On the same podium as two other students, who were afflicted with AIDS, Harry had recounted the ordeal of his past semester. When he reached and delivered his triumphant punchline—that he had just been awarded a Phi Beta Kappa key—he was accorded a standing ovation.

You might say that was Harry's last, and well-earned, hurrah. His condition immediately worsened. He missed the next three sessions, and when he finally called me, again from St. Vincent's Hospital, he sadly announced that the worst was true. He had just spoken to the oncologist who had told him how the cancer had so metastasized that it appeared to be infiltrating his kidneys.

I saw Harry just one more time. He came to see me soon after being released from the hospital. He briefly made it up the three flights of stairs. He could no longer come to therapy physically even if he wanted to. He pointed to his stomach. Underneath the T-shirt he was wearing, his stomach visibly bulged, a good three or four inches beyond what it had been just weeks ago. Yet, even if Harry could physically make it to therapy, he had made a decision to terminate therapy anyway. He spoke softly, hardly above a whisper, but with undeniable conviction. He had gotten everything he could from therapy. Now he had to make some major existential decisions which only he alone could make.

I listened, and then pointed out, as simply and effectively as I could, that while I would back whatever decision he ultimately arrived at, I, nevertheless, believed there were still benefits, especially given his condition, that therapy could give him. Respectfully, Harry shook his head no. I accepted with mixed feelings his decision: on the one hand, I felt guilty and upset that therapy and myself would be abandoning him in his final hours; on the other hand, there was a certain relief that perhaps the most stressful case I had ever experienced was coming to an end.

I said that perhaps, while everything else was slipping away, our relationship was the one meaningful area left upon which he could exert both choice and closure. It was my last interpretation, my final offering for what it was worth, and Harry seemed to accept it. It was the end of the session. He got up from the couch and slowly approached me. Solemnly and wistfully, he leaned over and shook my hand.

Five weeks later, I received a telephone call from his mother, who was in New York. Harry had died the previous afternoon. She had been with him at his deathbed, as had Susan—"the two people he loved most in the world."

Emotionally drained but lucid, his mother stayed on the phone with me for nearly an hour. She reminisced about her life with him, and recounted the steps leading to his death. Over and over again, she told me how much I and therapy had meant to her son, and that even in a short span of time she had observed significant changes in his ability to relate, especially to her. I responded by telling her how much I had learned from Harry and how, apart from that, it had been a joy just to behold and be in the company of such a scintillating, creative mind. "Yes," she cried, pleased and excited, "his mind *was* a joy to behold." She then asked if I had seen the obituary, appearing in the day's *New York Times*, written by Susan.

As soon as I got off the telephone, I reached for the *Times* and located Susan's obituary. In simple, beautiful language, it commemorated Harry as a priceless not-to-be-forgotten, lost love. Speaking for myself, I was sadder than I had expected. I wondered if, more than I realized, I had bought Harry's denial of his death and was somehow unconsciously expecting his gallant fight for life to never end.

At any rate, before I could effect my own closure with Harry, I had to make a decision. Should I or should I not attend his funeral? I felt strongly that by reminding me of the obituary, his mother was also inviting me to the funeral.

After some reflection, I decided my responsibility was still to my patient, Harry. By deliberately ending therapy in advance of the terminal stages of his illness, he was attempting to make his dying (at least as far as his therapist was concerned) a private, existential affair.

I decided I would respect that by not attending the funeral because I felt, as far as I could know, that that is what Harry had been telling me.

The Impact of Certain Death on the Psyche

Since artists are more narcissistic than most people, and since death is perhaps the ultimate insult and narcissistic injury (complete cancellation of existence), it is not surprising that Harry's principal defense, in the face of terminal illness, was denial. What did surprise me was the longevity and durability of his denial throughout the year that I knew him.

Elizabeth Kübler-Ross (1969) the eminent psychiatrist of

death and dying, has postulated five stages of reactions to terminal illness, the first being denial and the fifth, final stage supposedly being acceptance. Yet, in a year of working intensively with Harry—one of the most articulate, expressive patients I've known, who poured out his heart, especially during the last six months, upon every nuance of thought and feeling concerning the medical forecast of his death—he did not once get past, get unstuck from (or show any inclination to) that initial stage of denial. This was nowhere more in evidence, according to his mother's posthumous telephone conversation with me, than on Harry's deathbed: shot up with morphine to numb the pain and apparently successfully tranquilized, he was still periodically able to summon up, in the twelve hours preceding his actual dying, fits of truly defiant rage.

Not a whisper of resignation or acceptance of his death from Harry. Two other patients afflicted with major life-threatening diseases that I'd worked with intensively for a number of years—although neither were artists—displayed a similar inability to accept the fact of their very probable death manifested by a comparably powerful denial. As with Harry, there was plenty of anger and depression with these other two patients, but the overriding defense was denial.

Harry showed his denial in many ways. He repeatedly acted as though he were more medically astute than his doctors, and would grandiosely dismiss their interpretation of findings whenever it suited his needs. He insisted on leading his life, not only as if he were milking the present for everything he could before the inevitable end came, but as if he were rationally, soberly building for his future; that is, he spent a great deal of time in therapy trying to select the right graduate school that would give him the career base he needed to underwrite his projected, long-term playwrighting goals, while simultaneously laying a foundation for an ongoing relationship with Susan, which under any other circumstances, would have been convincing and real.

A patient's knowledge of terminal illness affects him in ways that other traumatic events seemingly do not. If there is greater denial of death, in order to protect one's narcissism from an unbearable insult, there is also greater self-love, greater narcissistic valuation of every facet of his life. Because everything is slipping away and is about to be lost, everything seems thereby more precious, and there is a sense of heightened drama as one hugs one's treasures to oneself for as long as possible. These patients become more empathic to the suffering of others, especially to the suffering of people who are similarly dying.

In this regard, I was often impressed by the expanded quality of Harry's empathy (far more than I had ever seen in him) for a friend who was in the last stages of AIDS. Each week Harry regularly visited him, bringing him soup, running errands for him, but, especially, trying to console him that the Karposi sarcoma (KS), the little purplish blotches appearing on his nose tip, cheeks, and ear lobes—were not as noticeably disfiguring as his friend feared they were.

For such patients, foreknowledge of their death may serve as a pardon from the consequences of small worries and thereby act as a buffer against anxiety, much of which, according to Freud (1926), is a signal to the ego about the possibility of important early danger situations being repeated in the immediate future. But death is the only anticipated event in our lives that has no future, and it may be that this sweeping cancelation of the space–time in which the multitude of small worries each of us is heir to are to be decided in, carries with it a necessarily energizing liberation. In other words, if you know you are going to die, you *also* know that thousands of the petty cares you have been obsessing about for much of your life cannot possibly materialize because there is not going to be sufficient time for them to materialize. Of course, there is the big worry, the big anxiety that one is going to die, especially that one is going to be dead; but despite that new massive concern, there is, nevertheless, an unprecedented letting go of countless, individual, lesser cares.

It is in this sense that knowledge of one's death can be perhaps the most meaning-laden experience of a person's life: something that functions, existentially, to prioritize one's life by almost automatically sweeping away everything that does not appear sufficiently meaningful. For such patients, a focus that may have previously been absent is dramatically added and foreknowledge of their death can serve as a kind of partial auxiliary ego.

Perhaps for such reasons Harry never seemed more psychologically healthy and never functioned better than when he was informed that he was terminally ill. This was also true for the patients I worked with who also had to contend with major, life-threatening diseases. They all mysteriously did better, it was almost as though knowing they were going to die was, somehow, therapeutic for them. One way to understand this, is by looking at death, not only as an external event against which the patient rails and reacts (Kübler-Ross 1969), but also an interaction (intrapsychic and interpersonal) between an extraordinary fate and a psychic constellation of defenses which meet in an unprecedented manner.

What are the ways in which foreknowledge of one's death impinges on the psyche, especially its defenses? While it has long been known how fear of certain death rouses defenses, it has not been sufficiently appreciated how it may also *strengthen* defenses. It can do this in two principal ways: by calling into play and activating the most adaptive features of the particular defense mechanism, or by alleviating or undoing some of the specific conflict which ordinarily elicits the defense mechanism in question. One such example of beneficial undoing (resulting in feelings of liberation) has already been given: the letting go of unnumerable petty cares and worries that simply do not make sense when stacked up against the big picture of death.

A different example, that of strengthening the defense, has been given by alluding to some of the ways in which narcissistic defenses (that is, defenses designed to maintain a healthy sense of self-esteem) are mobilized as never before once one is confronted with the ultimate and ugliest of narcissistic injuries.

If we turn to the area of neurotic, obsessional uncertainty (Freud 1909), we find an example of undoing naturally following from having knowledge of one's death. For if someone has a neurotic, obsessional need to relieve an underlying emotional ambivalence by establishing comforting compulsive rituals of concrete exactitude (e.g., counting), what greater substitutive gratification, what greater ritual of concrete certainty, can there be than the certainty of terminal illness? How can the ritual of obsessively numbering trivial things, for example, be compared in the psyche to the grandiose existential ritual of counting down the days to your own death? This was borne out by the fact that all of my dying patients upon receiving their diagnosis of terminal illness showed a general decrease in their past obsessive–compulsive behavior.

In terms of activating the adaptive features of a defense mechanism, *it might be said that the realization of actual concrete death to a certain extent (although not equally) can usefully mobilize every basic defense mechanism known.* The emphasis here, of course, is on the *can* because the realization of actual death can easily (and perhaps—on a statistical basis—more frequently) go the other way. That is, the abnormal stress and global anxiety triggered by knowing you are about to die, may overwhelm whatever defenses are raised against it; and instead of existentially heightened functioning, as in the case of Harry, there can just as well be a reverse sense of alarming annihilation, decompensation, and, perhaps, psychosis.

The outcome very much depends on whether the holding environment (Winnicott 1960) and the therapeutic alliance are capable of supporting the defenses enlisted to contain the traumatic threat of terminal illness. Since, as far as I can tell, Harry, as well as the other terminal patients I've worked with, dramatically elevated their level of functioning upon learning they were going to die, I believe the necessary favorable therapeutic environment had to be actively present.

Let us therefore look, from this admittedly specialized standpoint of a *favorable* therapeutic environment which at least has a chance of containing and holding up the dying patient, at some of the ways in which knowledge of one's death can strengthen, instead of wrecking, the psyche's defenses.

Take the case of the fairly sophisticated defense mechanism of intellectualization—the cognitive distancing, detachment, and attempt to symbolically manipulate whatever is perceived as irrational, disunited, disturbingly affective, or embarrassingly undeveloped. There is nothing I can think of that can so motivate the psyche to intellectualize as recognition that death (which means, above all else, death of the psyche) is imminent; and this was certainly borne out by Harry, who, although highly cognitive to begin with, rose to something of the stature of an amateur philosopher upon learning that a malignant tumor was buried in his brain.

It is no accident that the preferred philosophy of terminal patients is existentialism, even if they have never read a book on the subject. It can be understood the following way: historically, existentialism as a philosophy and as an applied method of psychoanalysis has endeavored to bring together three things that are not easily perceived as belonging together: the absolute certainty of our death; the seemingly unknowable distance separating us from our death; and the overshadowing, all-encompassing importance of that unique event, no matter how temporally nebulous. Much of the teachings of the great existentialists (Heidigger 1968; Sartre 1956) is a kind of urgent plea to live one's life as though the fact of death were luminously present and imbuing every transient moment with its transcendent meaning.

That they have to argue with such strenuous eloquence is testimony in no small part to the defense mechanism of denial; and, clinically, the fact of being confronted with a terminal illness, does incomparably more to overcome the instinctive, unconscious bias against accepting death than all the existential treatises in the world. This may be why—regardless of whether they have any particular philosophical talent, training, or education—the real existentialists are to be found, not in classrooms, but in cancer wards.

Another defense mechanism, much more primitive than that of intellectualization, is projection, which can be viewed as a kind of distancing away from the ego of whatever is perceived as anxiously invasive. Such projection is not only lateral, that is, from one person into another, but is also temporal—a thrust forward into the future. Freud's (1895) original metapsychological concept of thinking was that of a necessary, interposed delay between impulse and reality. According to this view, thinking was a cognitive trial-and-error experiment projected into the future to avoid the draining expenditure of having to carry out each and every impulse. By instead temporally representing the possible consequences of various permutations of intended actions, without being committed to faithfully living them out, thinking could save precious psychic energy.

However, in order for the mechanism of projection to be most useful in its designated Freudian role as a conserver of wasteful psychic energy, it is necessary not only to project up until the brink of the anticipated event, but to project *past* it. Instead of stopping before the intended event, projection should overshoot it, that is, it must move imaginatively through the anticipated event and beyond it, so as to cognitively look back on it and hopefully learn from it. A projection (as in the anticipation of one's own death) that carries you up until the brink of the event and no further is not much good (defensively).

That is like saying that there is a door marked X and behind it lies an event of unparalleled importance. You know you have to pass through the door, and once through every detail of your entire life will be permanently, radically altered. It is impossible not to want to know what the experience of that change will be like. It is impossible to accept or understand the traditional answer that no one has the slightest clue. It is impossible not to want to prepare and defend against so portentous an event that cannot ever pass through consciousness. But how to defend against an all-pervasive threat that seems completely unknowable?

Seen in this light, the defense mechanism of projection stands in a peculiarly ambivalent relationship to the realization of terminal illness. On the one hand, it is easy to see how the knowledge of imminent death bestows upon the future an importance it never had before and that therefore projection, as a defense mechanism, is correspondingly, enormously strengthened. On the other hand, the very purpose for which the defense of projection is brought into play—to project *past* the event so as to learn from it and cognitively absorb it—is effectively canceled by the nature of death.

As we saw from the case of Dan, paranoid defenses are built upon hypervigilance, the search for confirming clues, the anxiety about solving a mystery, and the need, above all, to uncover the whereabouts of one's enemy. What greater mystery is there than the mystery of what lies beyond life, and what could possibly whet the appetite for clues more? What greater threat or persecution than the knowledge life is about to be taken, and therefore what greater enemy than certain death? Knowing you are going to die, can place one in the ultimate paranoid–schizoid position (Klein 1946), and it can thereby mobilize paranoid defenses as never before.

Toward the end of his life, Freud (1938) discovered yet another defense mechanism, which he called splitting of the ego: it was a denial of reality, a kind of glorified having your cake and eating it, too, but one that was achieved at the price of doing structural damage to the ego (by splitting it). If we look at what happens upon realization of terminal illness, we also find a splitting of the ego. It is a splitting, not based on denial, but founded on reality. This splitting, of course, in the case of the dying patient, is between the present cumulative life forces and the threatened future cancelation of all those vital impulses and needs. The person who knows he will die shortly really does have one foot in life, in the here and now, and one foot out of life, pointed toward his projected death.

In this sense, it is a true existential split not based on denial. The existential split of a dying patient can be seen as between an ego of the present, and therefore of possibilities, and an ego of the future which is completely without possibilities—the quintessence of helplessness. In the case of the dying patient, the splitting of the ego, far from being a Freudian denial of psychic reality, is instead a genuine primordial process and actualization of an ineluctable, imminent reality. Very soon the ego will be split by death. It is not hard to see, in the dying patient, that this realization will be an irresistible spur and reinforcer of the more mundane defense of splitting of the ego.

Freud (1911) conceived of the ego as an intermediary agent and barrier between external reality and the id. Looked at this way, death represents the ultimate symbiosis, when external reality not only overcomes the barrier of the ego, but completely obliterates it. In death, external reality, far more than impinging on the internal private domain of the id, forms an unbroken, symbiotic unity with it. We are reminded of Sartre's great work on existentialism (1956) in which he envisioned death (what we are discussing from a purely psychotherapeutic standpoint) as the total exteriorization of the person—again what we would call the coming to pass of the complete absence of ego boundaries. To carry this a step further, we can see how knowing you are going to die can raise defenses generally employed against the threat of symbiosis, that is, defenses meant to uphold the boundaries of the ego and to reinforce a sense of identity and cohesive separateness.

If the fear of becoming symbiotic is at one end of the defensive continuum, the fear of becoming schizoid must be at the other. Typically, schizoid defenses protect against feelings of fragmentation, excessive and frightening isolation, unrealness, and annihilation of the self. They have been exhaustively catalogued by writers who dwell on the dividedness of the modern self (Bion 1977, 1990; Kahn 1981; Laing 1970; Searles 1960, 1979; Sullivan 1973). You do not have to be included in the class called schizoid to have made use of them at one time or another. They are available, in lesser degrees, to everyone. They are therefore certainly available in the case of the realization of terminal illness, when the ego must defend not only against the habitual psychic dread of self-decay, but against the impending, actual annihilation of the whole of the psyche.

Rationalization: Of all the defenses called into service by the realization of approaching death, this is one of the most susceptible. If the knowledge of death is truly the beginning of philosophy, it is natural when one comes face to face with, not the knowledge, but the actuality of death, to search for compensating, comforting (i.e., rational) thoughts. And when little in the way of concrete actions can be done, thinking—especially the defensive use of thinking called rationalization—is a powerful, appealing substitute. This was repeatedly shown by Harry: no matter how sick he became, no matter how discouraging were the results from his laboratory tests, he would usually come up with a fairly positive, rational way of regarding his situation.

Repression: Since this is a defense which deals considerably with the infantile past (Freud 1915), and since death is a uniquely occurring event with no antecedents, no past, and therefore no history, it does not come much into play. This is another way of saying the realization of terminal illness does not particularly trigger repression, because there is not anything particularly to repress (other than associated memories to sickness and death, such as attending funerals). If anything, the realization of terminal illness lessens and undoes repression, which was also borne out by my patients. After all, if repression is concentrated on the early past, and if death is surely going to obliterate that same early past, it follows that the recognition of impending death—with its promise of unparalleled forgetfulness—preempts, and to a corresponding degree, makes useless that very defense mechanism.

This points to one of the fundamental ways in which the defense mechanisms raised by the ego in the face of terminal illness are different. Traditionally, all the defense mechanisms, even Freud's (1926) signal functions of anxiety which is a residue of infantile danger situations, are based on the individual's psychic history and memory. Yet, the defenses raised by the ego, when there is knowledge of unavoidable, approaching death, are unique in that there is no individual memory of experiential history to draw upon. It may therefore be that what is *most terrifying and traumatic about death is not that it has no future (the most popularly voiced apprehension) but that it has no past.*

This means that the ego and its defense mechanisms, postulated on the derived expertise of a remembered, experiential past, are powerless against an event of which it has no memory.

Viewed this way, death represents the *absorption* of the ego and all its defenses; and since the ego, on at least this existential level, is totally defenseless against the arrival and passage of death, it may be why the denial of death is so powerful and difficult to eradicate. The ignorance of death, from this experiential vantage point of the psyche (the only one it really knows), is profound and complete.

The defenses that are raised, upon knowledge of terminal illness, are therefore different in at least this respect from all other defensive operations. Typically, defense mechanisms are employed to defend against the preparation and anticipation of an anxiety-producing occurrence, the arrival and passage of this same occurrence, and the projected consequences of the occurrence. By contrast, in the defense against certain death, you need only defend against the anticipation (putting aside posthumous concerns, such as a will, which are really defenses for others), not the occurrence itself or its consequences. There is therefore—if only measured against this temporal scale—*much less to defend*, which may be one more reason why such defenses can sometimes work surprisingly well.

That is one side of the coin. The other is that unless you work intensively with dying patients it is hard to appreciate the enormity, the near-impossibility of the defensive task which challenges them. For how can we defend against a momentous event if it is an experience we are never going to have (except perhaps for a fleeting, incipient moment)? How can we learn from an experience that never (so far as we are concerned) occurs and an experience that we can never remember? It can be summed up, from the standpoint of the double bind, this way: *the double bind of death is that the most important single event, affecting every experience of one's entire life, can itself never be experienced inasmuch as it is an event that cannot have a future (in the sense of projecting past the event), a present, and (perhaps most tellingly) a past.* Furthermore, the most frighteningly certain and indisputably real threat to the self—from the standpoint of being experienced—*is nonexistent* (when it comes, it comes with no footprints and no history).

It may be that part of the appeal of both conventional and unconventional religions is that they promise relief and escape from these profoundly troublesome double binds. Conventional religion, with its emphasis on the continuation of life after death, provides the missing future. Reincarnation, with its cavalcade of former existences, provides the missing past. And present-day paranormal investigations into reported out-of-body experiences of those who are pronounced medically dead, yet come back, provide the missing present.

According to Max Schur (1972), Freud's personal physician who attended him during some of his many agonizing cancer operations leading to his death, the founder of psychoanalysis believed that the concept of death did not exist in the unconscious. In terms of the clinical view being presented here, it is not hard to see that the acceptance of death (because it can never be based on an experience) must thereby differ from other acceptances inasmuch as it cannot be experienced as genuinely *real*.

This is not to deny there are truly religious people who are sincere in their faith. But the acceptance of faith (and I have worked with a number of such religious patients) is not at all the same thing as the acceptance of death, which is supposedly the absorption and integration into the psyche of *an experience*. The acceptance of faith is rather like the acceptance of a particular religious teaching, a principle and conduct of living; and the religious patients I've known—in terms of the experiential acceptance of death being discussed—did not differ in any important way from the nonreligious patients.

For all of these reasons, the classic denial of death may not be the stubborn pretence of ignorance in the face of the knowable (the basic scenario of the defense mechanism of denial), but a genuine manifestation and outcome of psychic helplessness which is the result of profound and total ignorance of just what the experience is that is supposed to be defended against. It is natural to simply turn away (deny) from something that cannot be seen, felt, experienced, remembered, or even convincingly imagined.

Of course, one can and often does project oneself into one's funeral or into the secret hearts of our posthumous friends. But this is a projection—unlike other future projections—that does not have a chance to ever be married to experience. Unlike other even fantastic projections (such as, for example, becoming President of the United States), there can be no conceivable reality reinforcement. Such projections, therefore, are more in the nature of fantasies and impossible daydreams (such as being able to fly like Superman), which may be why fantasies and daydreams, as defenses, are so powerful in terminally ill patients.

Seen this way, suicide can be, among other things, the denial of death inasmuch as it seems to envision death as a wished-for state: that is, something which it cannot be, a satisfying experience. Seen this way, the contemporary focus on acceptance of death, which in many ways I find admirable and necessary—if pushed to the extreme stage of postulating a final, so-called complete acceptance of death (Kübler-Ross)—*can itself become a denial of death.*

In summary: when there are favorable circumstances (in our examples, a very positive therapeutic alliance), the realization you are going to die can act like a massive adrenalin rush to the ego's basic defense mechanisms. By serving as a universal scapegoat and common enemy to all of the defense mechanisms, it can rally them as perhaps no other threat can. In so doing it can, thereby, automatically reinforce the basic function of the ego, which, according to Freud (1923), was to synthesize and collectively act on behalf of the psyche. This may be why, as I've observed and already mentioned, patients on the brink of death often dramatically raise their level of psychic functioning.

I began this chapter by saying how nothing is as painful for a therapist as to sit and watch your patient die. During the six months when it became absolutely clear that Harry was about to die, I repeatedly had to convince myself that there was something worthwhile in a relationship that basically revolves around one person trying to help another bear up best he can while everything materially, physically, and psychically precious leaks away.

That there was, in retrospect—in the context of everything seemingly being lost—such depth of meaning as experienced by myself, by Harry (and even posthumously expressed by his mother) was, ironically, one of the most affirmative instances of the benign power of therapeutic contact I have every encountered.

5
The Painterly Eye

Marie's Two Worlds

Of all the artists I've met and worked with over the past decade, there is one who symbolizes for me the essence of what I consider the artistic temperament, that is, someone who is blessed, or cursed, with a surcharge of runaway creative energy that cannot help but leave its stamp of originality on every part of the psyche that it touches.

That is another way of saying that even if Marie wanted to, it was hard for her to say, think, or feel something that was not at least in some way, original. As a therapist, my chief problem with her was to make sure I did not overly enjoy her sessions with me and to remind myself that—her delightful perceptions notwithstanding—my responsibility was to understand and to help her, if I could, and not to enthusiastically appreciate her.

Yet it was easy, even as a therapist, to slip into a passive audience role with her if only because she didn't even seem to be particularly trying to capture or engage my attention, and perhaps more importantly, because she was so full of surprises. By surprises I mean novel ways of perceiving and responding to her private world. For example, discovering in a corner of her courtyard a discarded, old-fashioned tin watering can; retrieving it like a buried treasure and transporting it to her apartment; and then—for about twenty minutes in the session—with amazing inventiveness, examining, extolling, and depicting an unsuspected multitude of visual aspects.

What made it memorable was that it did not seem pretentious, exhibitionistic, nor digressive, it was just her way of seeing things. And her way of seeing things with a painterly eye came naturally to her almost with the dawn of consciousness as a small child growing up in a rural section of Bridgeport, Connecticut. Everything she saw, from the Ingmar Bergmanian play of light and shadow in the winter woods, her studies of field animals (like a young Darwin), her fascination with encapsulated buds that unfurled on schedule in the spring, her admiration for the wonderful mechanical contraptions devised by her father, a failed inventor, which adorned the backyard of their house, were all seen through a stubbornly solitary, aesthetic purview.

She did not apologize for her division of her particular universe into an inner world, that to her was forever fabulous and always to be further explored, and an outer, mundane, depressingly dreary world she was condemned to inhabit with everyone else. For Marie it made perfect sense to conceive of her own world as being two worlds: that was not her problem. What was her problem was one of logistics—how to get from one place, one space to another without losing too much of herself along the way.

Space was a recurring theme and dominant metaphor in her therapy. There was the geometrical, visual space of the actual, concrete world. There was the less restrained, more playful space of her imagination, where she could juggle contours according to her aesthetic whimsy. There was the rigorous space of her oil paintings, where she would tax her creative powers to the fullest by posing and attempting to resolve difficult topological problems. And there was the space of her dreams in which not surprisingly, her conflicts were often geometrically represented: how to move from one level to another; how to escape a sense that the ground was realigning itself under her feet; how to find her way safely out of a terrifying labyrinth; how to rejoin two parts of a familiar object which, puzzlingly, had been torn apart.

Spatially, what was most exacting and baffling to Marie was what she considered her primary logistical and territorial problem. How to get from here to there. How to move her feet in the proper way so as not to bump into herself or into others in an unfamiliar, crowded, hostile street. How to read maps, memorize landmarks, and orientate herself, especially in an urban area of the compacted density of Manhattan.

In the early months of therapy, Marie devoted a good deal of time to what she labeled her "spatial dilemma." She recounted vividly her sense of horrified dislocation on the two occasions in her childhood when her parents, seemingly, abruptly, moved to a new neighborhood and a new house; how it took her months and months in the new place to recapture her former sense of herself. When she at last felt strong enough, as an eighteen-year-old, to relocate on her own terms—by moving into a friend's house in Los Angeles and joining a small enclave of eclectic artists—she experienced her first major trauma. It was a trauma that was geographical and spatial and not interpersonal, because her new artist friends were eager to absorb her, charmed by her demure, vibrant, yet slinky way of moving about, her unabashedly wide-eyed bewitchment at her surroundings, coupled with an undeniably original way of expressing herself.

What troubled and traumatized Marie, instead, was not the city but the newness of the city. Compared with Bridgeport, it felt like a foreign country, and compared with the ease she had acquired in her home town, she felt almost paralyzed in Los Angeles; for example, whereas she was an expert driver in Connecticut, she literally had to be shepherded by a friend and driven—even for a distance as short as several blocks—like an invalid.

Seven years later, Marie relocated a second time (to Manhattan), again moving into the waiting apartment of an accommodating friend, and again experiencing a similar trauma. Feeling petrified, dwarfed by the city, unable to conceive how she could ever walk safely in its streets, she promptly incarcerated herself in the apartment of her friend. For a month she refused to leave the premises at all, and when she did venture forth, for a long time, it was not without a chaperon.

It followed that someone for whom personal space was both precious and perilous would resist and defend to the best of her ability, hostile encroachments; and whenever Marie successfully did defend her turf (as she called it), especially if she did so courageously, she was justifiably proud. Sometimes too proud. There was the time she was awakened in her studio apartment in the early morning hours and discovered someone—having broken in through the window near the fire escape—in the process of vandalizing her apartment. Terrified, yet sufficiently enraged, she bolted from her bed, and lunged for the intruder whom she narrowly missed, and who managed to let himself out the front door. When I asked Marie what she thought she might have done, had she caught hold of the trespasser, she could only shake her head. She did not have an inkling of an idea. Her sense of violation had been so immediate and so painfully and uncontainably compelling, it left room only for reaction and not afterthought.

THE BRIDGE

Because Marie realized how much I genuinely appreciated her inner world (which she obviously loved to show me), I was able to point out how, perhaps, she had underrated the importance of the outer world—the second of her two worlds. I suggested that it might not be always expedient to adopt an either/or life strategy, to choose between a presumably, infinitely superior private world and a manifestly inferior, oppressively impersonal, public real world. There was another alternative which many people, including fine artists, favored: the creation of a personal bridge allowing one to travel at a preferred individual pace backwards and forwards whenever necessary between both worlds.

The metaphor of a bridge between two worlds, in the first year of therapy was a compatible one for Marie, appealing to her fondness for pictorial representation of her innermost feelings. It enabled me to explore with her in earnest her precious geometry of personal space and to eventually suggest—aesthetic considerations aside—that perhaps her division of reality into two worlds was itself a metaphor for a deeper division, that is, a schism between herself and others, between herself and her feelings, and even between one part of her mind and another.

Marie opened up after that. The interior landscape which she loved to talk about became progressively less abstract and more humanized. Topics she had regarded as pedestrian and therefore taboo—such as who was and who was not, who could be and who could not be a boyfriend—began to crop up. She was by her own admission, "shy" and the fact I was a man made it that much more difficult to discuss sexual matters. When she finally did get around to such personally delicate issues, she needed the crutch of fullblown irony and narrative humor. The odyssey of how she had lost her virginity was sprinkled with Salingerlike jokes meant to nostalgically recapture the poignancy and absurdity of adolescent folly.

Ten years later, at the age of twenty-eight, Marie still treated her love life as a subject more worthy of being lampooned than discussed. There were no men in New York: there were only gay men, married men, unavailable men, or cultural philistines. As she saw it, her history with men was a series of horror stories—a pattern of infatuation, disappointment, betrayal, and traumatic abandonment—leavened with comic interludes. Her accounts of former boyfriends were pieces of caricature rather than profiles: one whole relationship reduced to the unnerving memory of someone grinding his teeth in a hideously unsightly manner; another dismissed with the damning observation, "He didn't exactly have a mind that could cut through steel." When she finally did fall in love and believed she had found "the one" with whom she could have family and children, she was startled to discover that her designated husband had decided to devote his life to becoming a priest.

Without challenging her at times militant feminism, her stubborn sense of herself as "a strong woman," I was able to help Marie see what underlay her admittedly shaky judgment concerning the availability of men: that it had little to do with supposed deficits of femininity in herself, nor with characterological flaws of men as a group, but that it stemmed from her fragility, vulnerability, and detachment. Because she was so used to dividing her energies between her "two worlds," she had been unable to develop an animated connection to her true self. Simply put, in regard to men or relationships in general, she was never sure where she stood, what she felt, what she desired, or what on the most fundamental level she really thought.

Marie was twenty-eight years old when she first came to see me, and already she was bemoaning the subversive onset of "the big three-o." She felt confused, and wanted help in sorting out just about everything. The time she spent in her studio working on the oil paintings which she loved was being drastically cut in two by her new full-time job as a graphic arts designer, a euphemism for a mechanical draughtsman, a skill she was superb at, but felt was five levels below her real creativity. Well over a year had passed since her most recent boyfriend fiasco, and although she believed "manlessness" to go with the territory of being a discriminating, independent woman, she was worried about the growing possibility of remaining alone and unloved.

When therefore asked how it felt to confide in a man, she responded with a jovial, "You? You're my budzo." Budzo, it turned out, meant something harmless, likable, and avuncular—at least that is how she wanted me to be. She defended her habit of sometimes coining or making up new words, on the grounds she occasionally did not feel "like speaking English." That in itself was her joking way of saying she much preferred her own nonlinear, multilevel, creative way of seeing and expressing things to the linear tunnel vision of everyday language (and she frankly rejoiced when she happened upon James Gleick's *Chaos* [1987], a book she felt at last provided scientific respectability to her peculiar nonlinear way of viewing reality).

Partly because she so underrated her ability with language (which I, personally, found wonderfully original), she tended to overrate my own ability. So convinced was she that I had a way with words, that if I simply therapeutically mirrored what she had been saying in a brief sentence or two, she would react as though I had performed before her very eyes a minor miracle of language compression. Her admiration for my facility with language, as she saw it, was balanced by her sense that I was a bit of a Philistine in matters of art and taste. Once, letting her eyes rove along the interior of the office, she startled me by pronouncing, "This must be one of the ugliest rooms in the world—but, I don't know why, I like this dumb place."

Now, an interior decorator I'm not, but I felt the office decor was at least professionally adequate. The real reason the remark stung was because I felt betrayed by a patient with whom I imagined I had achieved an especially close therapeutic bond. On such occasions, Marie did not realize she was being nasty and biting, and instead saw herself as a salty, straight-shooting, strong woman.

That was one side of the coin. Underneath it lay a very tender dependency on me she was never quite able to acknowledge (because it was so frightening to her). This was driven home to me about eight months into the therapy, when—for the very first time and because of an unavoidable traffic jam—I arrived seven minutes late for the session. Although I carefully described the details of the traffic jam, was really sorry, and had done all I could to be on time, Marie was unable to recover from her initial shock that the one person in the world who was not supposed to abandon her had just done so. It didn't matter that an act of God had intervened: no excuse could ever be acceptable to her for my letting her down.

It showed me on a primary level how important and how

difficult it was for her to trust. Yet, because she trusted me as much as she did and felt she could say just about anything in therapy, she stayed four years. By that time, she had mastered what she believed to be a viable and fluid bridge between both of her worlds. More importantly, she had begun to consolidate a solid sense of a real true self and as a result felt considerably less disconnected, detached, and helplessly confused. She had even conquered her lifelong panic regarding travel and relocation and announced, upon termination of therapy (a bit counterphobically, I thought), that she was planning an adventurous trip around the world.

The Schizoid Artist

Once, when Marie was endeavoring, half-seriously, to psychiatrically diagnose her friends, I asked her how she would diagnose herself. She promptly replied "schizoid." It was interesting because although I would not personally have diagnosed her as clinically schizoid, and have worked with patients who were clearly more so, she nevertheless seemed to share and suffer from a number of characteristics prominently associated with so-called schizoid personalities. Since all of the artists I have worked with, to a greater or lesser degree, also exhibited some of these characteristics of alienation and detachment, I eventually came to the following conclusion (which I would now like to demonstrate): *that all other things being equal, the artistic temperament will greatly intensify, or bring out into the open, any latent schizoid tendencies (and we all have some) which exist in the psyche.*

There are many reasons for this. Artists are aware that because they are creative specialists, or freaks, depending on your point of view, that who they are and what they do is generally inaccessible to the overwhelming majority of people. Although they learn to expect this, their reaction is ambivalent: on the one hand, it can often feed their grandiosity that they are different and truly special in comparison with the ordinary run of people; on the other hand, it can work to reinforce their anxiety that they are somehow dangerously isolated, cut off from the mainstream of life in America, perhaps, even schizoid.

It is therefore easy for artists to feel, or to convince themselves, that there is something odd or different about them. As a rule, they do not readily perceive themselves as participating in the basic values of their society. They tend not to value security, steady social upward mobility, or career benefits, and as a result cannot realistically look forward to a pension nor count on the rewards and recognition that normally derive from pursuit of the traditional professions. Although there is a certain cultural respect that is perfunctorily granted to designated creative people in our society, artists come to realize how short-lived this can be if it is not accompanied by the standard, outward accoutrements of materialistic prestige and success. Another way of saying this is that the definition of an artist in America, unless it includes ample financial rewards, is a negative one.

An example of this was my patient Michael, a young actor who supported himself between jobs by working as a file clerk, and who one day, tired of being treated as just another menial, revealed to his co-workers that a year ago he had appeared in a major motion picture and actually acted alongside an internationally famous star. And for about a day or two, the magic of this accomplishment seemed to achieve its goal of differentiating him from the anonymity of being a file clerk. Yet, in just a few days' time, since in America you are pretty much judged by what you do, he was swiftly dragged back to earth with requests such as, "Oh, Michael, would you take this envelope and bring it to the third floor, please?" The schism between artist and society is not a one-way affair, and the public, for its part, can feel as alienated from the artist as the artist does from it. It is shown in the way artists are often thought of like technical wizards (physicists) or genetic prodigies (superstar athletes); that is, someone who seemingly naturally possesses some striking gift which is completely out of the realm of everyday experience, and to that degree is mysterious and incomprehensible. For this reason, people generally fail to grasp—and this is not to underrate the impressive motivating power of artistic inspiration—the artistic process as another type of evolutionary development and therefore almost completely misidentify with it. The creations of artists are viewed as wonders, things beyond the ken of normal human powers: such as seeing a man run twice as fast or jump twice as high as the average person. This is shown in the familiar question naively posed to artists, "How do you *think* of a symphony (or a novel)?"—as though a symphony or novel were a simple, direct flowering of an irrepressible and rare talent.

What is missing in this concept of the artist is the hard work that goes into even the most inspired creative process. Because of this, artists are not usually perceived as working or as working people. Curiously, artists collude in this misconception: since they themselves often view the most significant part of the creative process as inspiration—to be implemented in a heightened, flowing state—their actual hard work may not *feel* like work. Furthermore, artists are prone to perceiving nonartistic people as talentless drones, regardless of how brilliant or successful they are. It follows that artists have trouble perceiving themselves as working people, even working artists, and this is reinforced by the notoriously high overall rate of unemployment of artists. It is therefore easy for artists to resent the concept of working and the fact they are often economically driven to fall back upon humiliatingly noncreative survival work such as waitering (leaving them susceptible to additional double binds) can only make them more bitter.

Not surprisingly, either work inhibition or being creatively blocked is a major problem with artists. In ten years of working with artists, I rarely met one who either did not at some point suffer from an inhibition of work, or—if able to work—to some degree resent the fact. It is not uncommon for artists to perceive themselves as kind of glorified, aesthetic misfits. Time and again, as a therapist, I've heard, "There's nothing else I can do," as though their talent had castrated them and left them impoverished in all other vital areas of life. Painted into such a desperate corner, artists naturally find it hard to understand how such low-risk things as conspicuous consumption, long-term security planning, and traditional role-expectation can not only take precedence over creative self-actualization but be the dominating values in life. Finally, since they both want and perceive other people as passively accepting the role of audience, it is easy for artists to respond by trying to perform rather than by trying to be intimate. It is an arrangement reinforced by both sides: audiences also feel insecure and frightened to be intimate with such seemingly gifted people and therefore both need and find reassuring the security of guaranteed audience distance.

For all of which, artists are vulnerable to believing they are really defective misfits, incapable of being practically integrated into the society around them and therefore—at least in this fundamental respect—not whole people. It is not hard to see how, over time, this can lead to a feeling of being schizoid.

So far we have talked about the schism, on both sides, between artist and society. But what are the ways by which the artistic temperament, as an intrapsychic entity unto itself, breeds barriers to intimacy and lends itself to feelings of detachment and schizoid alienation?

Here are some of the most important ones.

1. Because artists both resist and resent work, they do not identify with the idea of developmentally fulfilling a role expectation. The result is they can feel cut off from the customary expectation of realization of normal roles: not just work and success, but as husband, lover, father, daughter, etc.

2. The artistic style of creation is a manic one: bursts of inspiration succeeded by spells of energized implementation which do not feel like normal work and seem alien to all other roles which by comparison appear to proceed by banal, serial steps. In this sense, artists can feel incomplete and alienated in regard to their capacity to fulfill normal roles.

3. Splits within the self: one part of the artist (creativity) is hyperdeveloped to the impoverishment of at least some other

parts of the rest of the psyche. We are reminded of Bion's (1990) description of the dilemma of the analyst who tries to keep pace with the runaway unconscious of a psychotic patient: he likened it to a lumbering consciousness pursuing a fast unconscious. To a certain analogous degree, artists can feel that the creative part of their mind is lightning fast and the rest of their personality, by comparison, is forced to spend an excessive amount of time trying to catch up. Because artistic creativity can be experienced as *an accelerated part of the psyche*, it can also seem split off and unintegrated with the rest of the mind, which again, by comparison, operates at a different and slower tempo.

4. As Marie often showed, artists can conceive of thinking as a nonlinear process which does not fit in with the structured, logical picture of reality typically presented by science. They are prone to experiencing their world in a disorderly, discontinuous, and nonlinear way, a process that dramatizes affects and thoughts that appear to emerge or erupt helter-skelter from the core unconscious as opposed to the more computerlike activity of their conscious cognitive mind. In a reverse sense to Ernst Kris's (1950) concept of regression as being in the service of the ego, artists may consider their cognitive linear thinking to instead be in the service of their dynamic, nonlinear creativity. And as such artists are *vulnerable to feeling schizoid in their very thought processes*: because the bursting of creativity from their unconscious is more pronounced, they are more or less forced to experience the division between their unconscious and conscious as also more pronounced (or discontinuous).

This discontinuity cannot readily be brushed aside nor denied by artists. Since creativity principally comes from the unconscious, and since flashes of creative inspiration are often so compelling, artists may justifiably feel they periodically make direct, vivid contact with their own unconscious. It is analogous to the experience of dreaming of nonartistic people, with the significant exception that the creativity of artists cannot be simply sloughed off, compartmentalized, and relegated to a physiological, dreaming part of the brain.

Accordingly, artists are stuck with and have to *feel* the split between their unconscious and their conscious, and find it difficult not to include it in at least a part of their regular self-perception. Because creativity and the unconscious are thereby, if only partially, integrated into the fabric of everyday, waking reality, artists may not have *as seamless a sense of the unity of the mind* as other people, where contact with the unconscious is more minimal and can be treated as an epiphenomenon (dreaming). And that, of course, can contribute to feeling schizoid.

5. The analogy between creative inspiration and therapeutic interpretation: creative inspirations of artists resemble interpretations made by therapists in as much as they make the unconscious conscious—but the connections are aesthetic ones, like trying to tie together the pieces of an artistic puzzle. It is not sufficiently appreciated how much *insight* is involved in artistic inspiration. Not insight (from a therapist) couched in cognitive reflections concerning maladaptive behavior, but insight into long-standing technical barriers and artistic problems. Creative inspiration on the one hand can seem more powerful and more truly symbolic of unconscious processes inasmuch as it appears to come, when it does come, of its own volition and is not invoked from without (sometimes fostering the paranoid suspicion that the unconscious contents are not really there but were *put* there by the sorcerer's hand of the analyst). Generally, an interpretation given by a therapist will involve more working out on the part of the patient in order to integrate the insight (again, provided by the therapist) with feeling and other aspects of the patient's personality. By contrast, the creative insight of an artist, even though it carries with it the mandatory and sometimes agonizing task of actualizing the inspiration, seems to emerge in an already more completed and integrated form. This may be—to compare it with an interpretation offered by a therapist—that since all the work has been done without outside help, the synthesis that does emerge into consciousness is necessarily more finished than the insight which arises through the external agency of a facilitating therapist. This may be why the creative inspiration of an artist can bring with it

an immediate, undeniable power to capture and enlist the ego's approval. There is therefore much less *resistance* on the part of the artist to his own creative insight (usually assent is quickly given) than there is in the case of the therapist endeavoring to induce insight through interpretation of a patient's unconscious, where resistance is more often the rule rather than the exception. From the standpoint of the double bind, the double bind of interpretation is this: that what should only meaningfully emanate from the deepest, most personal, autonomous core of the unconscious can only come from outside the person.

There is another paradox here. While on the one hand the artist's unconscious does more work for him by producing more finished, synthesized insights, there is simultaneously imposed on him the heavy burden of implementing these beautiful inspirations. And here is where the inhibition of the capacity to work, the resentment of working, and the inability, as shown by Marie, to move from the inner to the outer world, come into play. Artists are therefore people who go through life being presented with a series of visions, small or large, which are like potential dreams-come-true just waiting to be fulfilled. Yet, it is just this impairment of the pedestrian but crucial step-by-step working out process, the confusion as how to transpose the inner onto the outer, which, ironically, in the artist leads not only to feelings of frustration but also to a real sense of being split in a schizoid way.

Such feelings of being schizoid in both artist and nonartist, have traditionally been treated as the products of developmental warps (Sullivan 1973) or failures of the early maternal facilitating environment (Winnicott 1965). Around 1940, a picture of the so-called schizoid personality began to be built up, modifying the previous psychoanalytic model of repression followed by symptom formation, and eventually became one of the dominant clinical configurations of our time. Fairbairn (1940) provided perhaps the first, and still valuable, phenomenological account of schizoid factors in the personality. He spoke of the overemphasis and obsession with an inner reality, the presence of "splits" in the ego; the depersonalization of the object (person) and the deemotionalization of the object relationship. He also singled out the peculiar difficulty schizoid people experience when it comes to emotional giving, and their deployment of a technique of playing roles as a defensive substitute. It was Fairbairn who pointed to the importance of secrecy and the nursing of a secret superiority (like a Mona Lisa smile) often noted in the schizoid personality, and its complementary side—the "plate-glass effect"—wherein the schizoid is terrified his carefully contrived defenses are actually transparent.

Helene Deutsch (1942) added to the picture with her well-known conception of the "as if" personality with the bizarre "staged" quality of its relationships. The great British psychoanalyst D.W. Winnicott (1958) described the excessive passivity and compliance of the schizoid personality with its elaboration of a defensive false self meant to hide the more fragile true self, which in turn, suffers the fate of being unable to experientially develop. Winnicott's disciple, Masud Khan (1974), expanded on the pioneering researches of his teacher and took special note of the psychic deficits which are the price of erecting schizoid defenses. Khan speculated that the schizoid personality, because he can not face the true source of his anxiety, transforms it into pain and, in effect, becomes a "pain addict," hiding the underlying sense of deadness, emptiness, and derealization and providing (via the immediacy of pain) a pseudo sense of intactness of the ego. Khan further speculated that the ego-ideal as such is not an introject but a psychic substitute standing for the lack of an early primary object (usually the mother); that schizoid personalities typically want but fear a regression to their dependency; and that their random defenses revealing only aspects of a self-experience are not the result of repression but are true examples of the missing pieces of a fragmented reality.

Suppose now, instead of looking at whatever features of schizoid development there are in artists as the product of failure of the early maternal facilitating environment—although there is plenty of that to be observed in their childhood history—we turn things around and try to imagine the impact and effect which the unique constellation of characteristics called the artistic temperament may itself exert upon the rest of the psyche—especially its capacity to elicit the aforementioned clinical signs of the so-called schizoid personality. If we do that, an interesting picture of reciprocal interaction emerges.

The Disappointing Real World

The artist, because of his excess of creativity and abnormally charged imaginative life, is naturally preoccupied with his inner world. Such inward retreat does not have to be bolstered (although it can) by the defensive need to hide and withdraw from the real world, which is a common feature of the schizoid personality. Over the course of time, the inner world of the artist can gradually evolve to a sufficiently disproportionate degree that an unmistakable discontinuity or schizoid split—by comparison with the unimaginative, outside factual world—can easily arise. In artists, the plate-glass effect alluded to by Fairbairn may actually exist, but in a reverse way: artists, because they are misunderstood by the public at large, tend to feel they are opaque, not transparent. By contrast, they often regard other people as unimaginatively, factually simple and thereby transparently understood. If we pursue Fairbairn's plate-glass metaphor, it is more accurate to say they view themselves as looking out upon the world through the privilege of a one-way mirror.

It is therefore natural for the artist to imagine he is privy to a secret superior world that is beyond the grasp of the average person. Although artists often deny their dependency (as Marie did) the fact they typically find themselves at a socioeconomic disadvantage will force them into more postures of compliance than they would like. The "as if" personality of Helene Deutsch can come rather easily to artists who have a certain dramatic flair and sometimes cannot help but dramatize whatever happens to them—which, in turn, adds a theatrical aspect to their personal relationships. In the case of artists, this may not only be (as in schizoid as-if people) the need to dramatize so as to cover up inner deadness, but the consequence of having an eye for the dramatic ingredient and naturally perceiving what is legitimately theatrical about the real world.

Because of this, artists are likely to regard the concrete, public world as *not* real in the sense it does not ring true on the dramatic level. Since artists tend to search for, and find satisfying, dramatic cohesiveness in the real world (which by definition, lacks just this quality), and not linear, concrete cohesiveness, they are constantly reduced to experiencing the world as dramatically implausible, false, and finally absurd. And in this sense the world does not appear real. Another way of saying this is that artists are continually disappointed in the real world and do not understand why it has allowed itself to get into such dramatically and aesthetically poor shape. The consequence of the artist's sense of the dramatic meaningless of the everyday world can be indistinguishable from the often noted schizoid feeling of *derealization.* To sum up: *if the world does not appear dramatically, aesthetically plausible and convincing to the artist, then, to a corresponding degree, it can seem unreal and schizoid.*

Depersonalization: The abnormal creativity of the artist can act as an inadvertent aesthetic filter or censor between itself and the world, between taking in the world and responding to it. The artist may thereby operate under a heavy burden of imposing some dramatic sense on his life and actions which in turn can create an additional delay between perceiving and reacting that the nonartist does not have to experience. Again, inadvertently but powerfully, it can contribute to the delay or disconnection between feeling and response that is a classic diagnostic sign of schizoid personality.

A sense of depersonalization, of object relationships being staged or rehearsed (as in schizoids), may follow. The artist because he feels a greater need than other people to impose a dramatic, aesthetic order upon his life, may have more trouble responding in a banal, uninteresting way and therefore require more time to shape behavior in a dramatically meaningful way. *Since the artist needs not just to behave but to creatively behave—and since this is extraordinarily hard to do on everyday basis for everyone, including gifted artists—what comes across as stilted, theatrical staginess (as in schizoid personalities) may be the inevitable failure of someone trying to do an impossible task: impose dramatic order upon daily life.*

Finally, the *false self* compliance of the artist is a protective shield which hides the true self. It may be the nature of the true self (Winnicott 1955) in the artist *needs* to be hidden because of the real splits that exist between it and society at large; and the tendency to hide the artistic true self may not arise from early maternal deprivation but from a much later perception of the lack of society's attunement to the true self of the artist. The effect, of course, is the same. The artist, from a long history of hiding and needing to hide the true self, can experience himself as schizoid. An anxious compliance—the sense the real world has little use for the artistic true self unless packaged in brazenly successful, concrete terms it can understand—follows automatically from this.

To summarize once more: all other things being equal, the artist is more liable than the nonartist to experience himself as schizoid.

6
If Wittgenstein Were a Patient

THE TORTURED YOUNG PHILOSOPHER

The existential philosopher, William Barrett (who was my former teacher), once remarked, in a literary reminiscence (1982), that the most intelligent man he had ever met was the critic Lionel Trilling. If I were asked to make a similar designation, I would without question nominate the great philosopher Ludwig Wittgenstein, someone I've encountered and feel I know (although I have not met personally) through the process of becoming and being a devoted and enthusiastic student for many years. What I respond to and think I appreciate in Wittgenstein—although I am neither a philosopher nor logician by training—is this: an almost magical ability to retrieve from a single sentence, a brief phrase, or a traditional line of inquiry a seemingly flawless distillation of original pure thought. What's more, such golden nuggets of thought were often clothed in Wittgenstein's famous aphoristic and enigmatic prose style—a style that rightly has earned him a place among the modern masters of German prose.

I mention Wittgenstein in the context of this book, first, because he was perhaps as much of an artist as he was a philosopher; and, second, because—although he has been academically scrutinized and exhaustively studied—no one, so far as I know, has written about him from the less esoteric, more personal, psychoanalytic perspective. Part of this omission has to be attributed to the efficacy and force of Wittgenstein's wish: he deliberately drew an opaque curtain of silence around his life, his innermost thoughts, and, especially, his feelings. He even elevated this imposed silence to the stature of a philosophical canon: whatever could not be spoken properly and clearly, should not be expressed (be kept silent). It accounted in no small part for his celebrated reputation of having a "dark" side—a mysterious, brooding, perhaps mystical dimension to his personality.

As a psychoanalytic psychotherapist I could not help but speculate on this dark side and wonder what possible light therapy—had Wittgenstein ever consented to being a patient—might have added. I realized that so great was Wittgenstein's antipathy to close encounters of any kind, that even a Freud would have found it difficult, if not impossible, to therapeutically engage him even for the briefest of times.

From all accounts, Wittgenstein was a profoundly guarded man whose pervasive suspiciousness of human contact turned him into something of a perpetual social recluse. It seemed likely, therefore, that his distinctive, powerful personality would have interacted with his creative genius in a dynamically interesting way and that a psychoanalytical examination of such connections would prove meaningful. In his famous study of Leonardo da Vinci, Freud (1910)—setting careful constraints on his own methodology—warned that the most psychoanalysts could ever hope to attain in such an investigation was an understanding of the underlying psychopathology and *never* an explanation of the creative act of genius.

To attempt a psychohistory of a contemporary figure of Wittgenstein's stature would be not only intrusive, but irreverent. But to consider on a cognitive basis how his personality—along lines, for example, suggested by David Shapiro in his classic study *Neurotic Styles* (1965)—might have informed, infused, nudged, or even partially contributed to his creative output seemed both worthwhile and justifiable.

Having so decided, I confided my ideas to my friend, a very intelligent and sensitive woman, whose first reaction was to inwardly cringe (she was too kind to outwardly cringe). She immediately wanted to know if he had any direct heirs, and I told her I was certain he did not, and I very much doubted if there were any indirect heirs. I then relayed my intent to connect Wittgenstein's well-known paranoid style of relating with certain equally well-known idiosyncrasies of his published work; and my friend did not bother to hide her annoyance. Paranoia was a horrible word and to say someone, even if it were true, was paranoid was therefore in some way to brand him with a stigmatizing label. I pointed out that to say someone had a cognitive paranoid style was not at all the same thing as saying he was clinically paranoid; that I, personally, consider paranoia to represent a deficiency of relating that is sad rather than horrible; and that thinkers such as W. W. Meissner (1978) believe the so-called paranoid process is a universal feature of human development.

Therefore, the Wittgenstein that is presented here is the man for whom human intimacy, from every published report, was problematical and potentially treacherous. It is a style of relating that I've encountered, in one form or another, time and again in my patients. It is a style of relating that has been observed in Wittgenstein by many people, but has never—so far as I know—been psychoanalytically connected to his published writings. Which is why I include him.

Wittgenstein's story extends from Vienna—the cultural matrix and catalyst for Freud, Wittgenstein, and geniuses as diverse as Arnold Schoenberg, Karl Kraus, and Moritz Schlick (Janik and Toulmin, 1973)—to Cambridge where the young, undergraduate

Wittgenstein will meet, join minds, (and then bump heads) with the likes of Bertrand Russell, G. E. Moore, and Alfred North Whitehead. From the start he is an iconoclast, his iconoclasm indulged in by established, world-famous intellects who are taken aback by the dazzling force of both his mind and his personality (Barrett 1979). Afterward, Bertrand Russell would say that he learned more from his young student, Wittgenstein, than he was able to teach him; and he prophesied that it would be this same student who would provide the next turning point in philosophy (Barrett 1979, p. 33).

The prophecy is an inspired one. Beginning with Russell and Whitehead's recently published, epoch-making *The Principia Mathematica* (1910) wherein they attempt to reduce the entire world of mathematics to the laws of logic to guarantee its certainty, Wittgenstein goes on, at age twenty-nine, to produce a work so revolutionary that it is destined to change the course of Western philosophy. *The Tractatus Logico-Philosophicus* (1922), in many ways, is an extension of the sweeping program of mathematical logic ushered in by Russell and Whitehead. But it is much more. A radical who will not stop short of the final step, Wittgenstein takes the ideas of Russell and Whitehead and applies them to all of language. He imagines what the world would be like if it could be expressed purely, simply, and completely in logical form. He does not shrink from the daring conclusion he is led to: the world is the totality of all facts, and these facts have a special relationship, or lack of relationship to one another. "Any one fact can either be the case, or not be the case, and everything else remains the same" (*Tractatus*, 121, p. 31). Wittgenstein is picturing a world so supremely disembodied and disconnected, that the existence or nonexistence of any particular fact makes no difference whatsoever. It is a world in which the hegemony of logic— the truth or falsehood of any particular fact—is made perfect. So perfect that he can actually claim, "the truth of the thoughts communicated here seems to me unassailable and definitive" (*Tractatus*, p. 29), and conclude, "the problems have in essentials been finally solved" (*Tractatus*, p. 29). But the problems that have been solved are problems of logic. At the closing of the *Tractatus*, in a strange mystical turn, Wittgenstein suddenly says, "Whereof one cannot speak, thereof one must be silent" (7, p. 187).

THE MYSTERY OF THE UNSAID

One wonders what it was that lay wrapped in Wittgenstein's silence. It seems to include much if not all of what would normally be called emotional, passionate, sexual, moral, mystical, ethical, meaningful. Logical positivists, inspired by the starkly logical world pictured in Wittgenstein's theory of language, chose to overlook the meaning and enormity of his silence. While existential philosophers like William Barrett (*The Illusion of Technique*, 1979) will make much of it, for our purposes, it is enough to show, now, that from the outset of his philosophical career, Wittgenstein was a divided man: the rebelliousness and opposition he aims at his mentors, Whitehead and Russell, have, in some puzzling but deep way, been also internalized.

This ambivalence is so pervasive that it applies even to his most cherished ideas. On the one hand, the *Tractatus* will take the mathematical logic of Whitehead and Russell, and elevate it to an unprecedented height; on the other, it will simultaneously plant the seeds of ideas that will eventually overthrow it. Wittgenstein does this by introducing his now famous truth tables: he wants to show the tautologous character of logical statements. By employing the truth tables, he can tabulate the various possibilities of truth and falsehood for any component part of a proposition in logic and by demonstrating that the result for the whole, in whatever case, will always be true—prove this tautologous character. Another way of saying this is that the proposition of logic is true whatever the facts may be. Therefore, it can say nothing about the world. The logical proposition, "Either it is a, or it is not a" will always be true, regardless of the actual state of a. Therefore, it can tell us nothing about a (or the world).

This is a crucial point in the *Tractatus*, when Wittgenstein begins to subvert the sanctity of the mathematical logic he himself is championing, by calling it, at bottom, tautologous. From here, it is but a succession of steps until the later *The Blue and Brown Books* (1958) and the posthumously published *Philosophical Investigations* (1953), works in which Wittgenstein seemingly will reverse most of the spirit, method, and results of the *Tractatus*. Wittgenstein's "reversal" has been described (Pears 1969) as a dramatically rare change of mind in the history of philosophy. Looked at from the angle of logical consistency in the history of ideas, it does stand out as unusual. But looked at from a different angle (the psychoanalytic one), the apparent lacuna in logical consistency may be explained—as is sometimes the case in analytic investigations—by unconscious determinants. The two celebrated, contrary Wittgenstein philosophical positions—logical atomism epitomized in the *Tractatus*, which helped launch logical positivism, and the seemingly antilogical, behavioristic, ordinary language movement presented in the equally influential *Philosophical Investigations*—psychoanalytically compared, show enough correspondence to suggest, if not a reaction formation, at least a compromise formation. To put it one more way, two radically and apparently disparate philosophical positions show surprising underlying unity.

The similarities are (1) both rely exclusively on language as the final reference point, and stop there; (2) both view the world essentially through the prism of language; (3) both effectively shut out affect and dynamic personal meaning; and (4) both are radically uncompromising, all-or-nothing in their supposedly antithetical viewpoints.

The differences are also revealing. Wittgenstein, in his later phase, seems as obsessed with flexibility as he was originally with orderliness and logical consistency. Again and again, in *Remarks on the Foundations of Mathematics* (1956) and *Philosophical Investigations* (1953), he lashes out against the tyrant of "necessity" and "the logical must." Instead of the truth tables of the *Tractatus*, he inserts the hegemony of what he will call "language games" and ordinary usage. In this second philosophical position Wittgenstein, typically, goes all the way. He uses his genius to try to show how even the hallowed, logical law of the excluded middle—a thing can not be itself (*a*) and not itself (not *a*) at the same time and in the same place—may be undermined: "Why should Russell's contradiction not be conceived as something that towers above the propositions and looks in both directions like the Janus head?" (as quoted in Barrett 1979, p. 111).

Here Wittgenstein is being perversely provocative, but he is also being quite serious. More and more, he seems to fight bitterly against a persecutory sense of unbearable rigidity and authoritarian confinement that more and more seems (to us) internally located. Wittgenstein, himself, places the blame for his philosophical anguish elsewhere: on the misapplication of crossed metaphors, on the lack of appreciation of ordinary language usage, on the overvaluation of mathematical logic, on inherent subtle flaws in the nature of thought, language, the mind itself. He looks everywhere except within himself. According to our thesis, a study of the relationship between Wittgenstein and psychoanalysis, we might summarize this point by saying that *Wittgenstein, who in terms of linguistic analysis, penetrated more deeply than anyone—in terms of the psychoanalytic psyche—stayed always on the surface.*

Philosophers like Barrett, wishing to gain conceptual access to Wittgenstein by means other than mathematical logic and analytic philosophy, have speculated on the possible meanings of his celebrated "silence." Barrett indicates Wittgenstein was a deeply ashamed homosexual (1979, p. 66) and suggests this may have been an important personal ingredient in his philosophical persona of forever suffering, endless searching. Whether this is so, what there does seem to be—and this notwithstanding the traditional abstract impersonality of philosophical writing—is a curtain of silence drawn tightly over the slightest hint of personal sexual orientation. It is not that Wittgenstein is shown to be without passion and love; on the contrary, he is presented (Von Wright and Malcolm 1958) as fiercely passionate, but it is a Socratic passion, only for the truth.

Wittgenstein showed, as perhaps no one else in this century did, how there could be such a thing as a *trauma of language.* Time and again, he illuminates the painful, endless confusion, the hopeless knots that abuse and misuse of language could bring about as symbolized in the so-called great philosophical problems (which he originally believed he had solved). He set as his goal to let the fly out of the bottle. He was talking about language and its conceptual agonies in its purest form, but in our view, he was also talking about himself. Looked at psychoanalytically, Wittgenstein appears to use his philosophy as a highly sophisticated defense against his id. By drawing a philosophical veil around himself, effectively closing off all personal meaning and affect, Wittgenstein is also using language to *shut out the world*. A curious offhand but telltale sentence, occurring in *Remarks on Color* (1977), perhaps illustrates this well. In a typically Wittgensteinian passage about the expression, "I see," the philosopher matter-of-factly says, "People on the street often take me for blind" (p. 54e). To us the effect is eerie (all the more so because it is delivered so drily, so philosophically, so unself-consciously). We can only wonder at the intensity of disconnected inwardness that could regularly elicit so gross a perceptual distortion.

David Shapiro in his study of neurotic styles (1965) devotes a chapter to the paranoid style. Describing the general behavior mode of the paranoid, he finds crucial: a certain "continuous, tense and antagonistic directedness, intentionality, purposefulness; 'operating'; general aim is defense against threat" (p. 106). Everything we have by his own hand, or those closest to him, strongly suggests Wittgenstein possessed an abundance of these characteristics. He is tense, antagonistic, willfully intentional, forever guarding against threat—to the extreme. He finds fault and reasons to distance with everyone. In the first year of their friendship, Wittgenstein sends a letter to his great mentor, Bertrand Russell, advising him they can never be friends: their values are too far apart (Barrett, p. 33). In his private classes, according to Malcolm (1958, p. 27), Wittgenstein is a "frightening person": "Once when Yorick Smythies, an old friend of Wittgenstein's, was unable to put his objection into words, Wittgenstein said to him very harshly, 'I might as well talk to this stove'" (p. 27). He is morbidly irritable, suspicious of everyone: he meets the mathematical physicist Freeman Dyson, then an undergraduate, and when Dyson, out of politeness, inquires as to the nature of his studies, Wittgenstein grows wary—wanting to know if Dyson "is a journalist" (Malcolm 1958, p. 65). There are other traits Wittgenstein possessed (also mentioned by Shapiro): he is peculiarly nonsensual; talks about becoming a monk and manifests "an intense desire for purity" (Malcolm, p. 71); he is pathologically unstable. Three of Wittgenstein's brothers committed suicide, and according to his student and friend G. H. Von Wright (Barrett, p. 66): "It is probably true that he lived on the border of mental illness. A fear of being driven across it followed him throughout his life."

Turning from the general behavior mode of the paranoid to the mode of attention, Shapiro describes it as "extremely acute, intense and narrowly focused; fixed on its own idea, searching only confirmation; biased; characterization suspicious" (1965, p. 105). He elsewhere describes the paranoid style as one of psychological bias (the opposite of suggestibility) that can willfully impose its own conclusion anywhere; that loathes surprises. Although not intended to be, it is an apt description of Wittgenstein's style. To anyone who has not seriously studied him, it is difficult to convey a proper sense of the abnormal, almost obsessed focus of his writing. William Barrett, himself a distinguished American philosopher, commenting on the fact Wittgenstein hammered out his first great landmark philosophical work while actively serving as an infantryman in the First World War, says: "That a work so concentrated and compact in form should have been conceived and brought to completion amid the life of the trenches cannot but fill us with awe at the intensity of mind of the thinker himself" (p. 34).

ESCAPING FROM THE PARANOID STYLE

Let us look at Wittgenstein's writing and thought—psychoanalytically, not philosophically—and conceive of it as a cognitive, paranoid style following David Shapiro (1965). A somewhat different but interesting perspective emerges. We can see Wittgenstein's early yearning to construct a consummately logical language, as a paranoid attempt to cleanse his private conceptual universe of every irritant and impurity he cannot personally control. Seen this way the *Tractatus*—apart from its philosophical destiny—is also a personal, extraordinarily single-minded attempt to close off and fend off the world without. Seen this way, his celebrated silence—"Whereof one cannot speak, thereof one must be silent"—apart from laying down the logical rules for what can and what cannot be said meaningfully, is also a repressive barrier to the world within. Because of the narrow focus and willful search only for confirming clues, Shapiro notes (p. 65) there is in the paranoid style a loss of a sense of proportion resulting in a loss of the world. The loss of the world in its fuller, richer proportions takes the form (in the paranoid style) of a rigid, obsessive craving for certainty; a severe restriction of the inner, sensual, affective world, and a consequent preference for mechanical objects, mechanical schemes, mechanizations of all kinds. What greater certainty is there than in Wittgenstein's early logical atomism, his attempt to structure a universally perfect, totally logical language? What greater lack of surprise, than in the gloomy, tautologous world of the *Tractatus Logico-Philosophicus* where "any one fact can either be the case, or not the case, and everything else remains the same"? What greater example of the mechanization of thought and language in the history of philosophy, than Wittgenstein's great masterpiece, the *Tractatus?*

What Shapiro does not include in his study of the paranoid style is the element of genius. *It may be that the bizarre conjunction of profound originality, of first rate genius, and pronounced (perhaps pathological) paranoid style creates much of the tension that goes into his unique, oracular style.* There has probably never been anyone in the history of philosophy who has written with such breathtaking originality, such wholehearted, vibrant feeling on a subject traditionally so clear-cut and lifeless as logic. In the light of such tension, we see Wittgenstein, on the one hand driven by his paranoid style, fashion an airtight, rigidly perfect, logical prison (personified by the *Tractatus*); and on the other, propelled by flights of imagination like a philosophical Houdini, execute his wonderful escapes.

Wittgenstein's small book *On Certainty* (1969) shows this. Again and again, with unbelievable concentration and patience, we see Wittgenstein—almost animal-like—circling and trying to close in on his single, abstract prey, in this case, certainty. It is easy to say that Wittgenstein, like a good paranoid, is scanning his private terrain for a safe avenue of approach (Shapiro 1965). But what is wondrous in the case of our philosopher—whether his particular search for certainty has overtones of a paranoid style or not (and we believe it unmistakably does)—is how fruitful that search is. Wittgenstein appears seduced by his own genius: a fairly commonplace, intellectualizing, paranoid suspiciousness and craving for certainty, joined and elevated by genius, repeatedly leads to findings of philosophical beauty. With such reinforcement it is understandable he will press forward, not backward. With such reinforcement, it is understandable that he will not pause to consider whether it is solely his genius that leads him to believe the philosophical answers he proposes are "unassailable": but that perhaps it is also his *need* to be "unassailable," to be perfect, to be absolutely right. Because of this, part of our fascination with Wittgenstein may be our fascination at *seeing a genius, literally, trying to think his way out of despair*. Analysts know better than anyone that it can't be done, not even by Wittgenstein.

WITTGENSTEIN AND PSYCHOANALYSIS

If we now compare Wittgenstein and his use of language and psychoanalysis and its use of language, some immediate, substantial differences arise. First of all, if analyst and analysand were ever to conform to Wittgenstein's exquisitely exact, logical standard of what can and what cannot be meaningfully said, very little of what goes on in the consulting room would be sayable. It is not that psychoanalysis denies the importance or results of linguistic analysis, it just places a far greater emphasis on the possible latent, personal, or motivational meanings that may be condensed in the more manifest logical confusions or mistakes. This would extend especially to the more gross, logically self-contradictory, tautologous, or meaningless verbalizations contained in thought disorders. Whereas the approach of Wittgenstein to language could be said to be more analytic, the approach of psychoanalysis could be called much more projective (psychologically). In a sense psychoanalysis, regarding language, begins where Wittgenstein leaves off. In contrast to Wittgenstein who often seems to be restraining, purifying, and delimiting language, psychoanalysis widens the range of language, mainly by *spreading* the network of personal meaning which it does by listening for and discovering unsuspected, hierarchal levels of meaning.

In contrast to Wittgenstein who found so much of what was said unmeaningful and would sometimes speak of the man who was *meaning blind, there is no meaning vacuum in psychoanalysis*. As analysts, we know there is no verbalization or psychic manifestation so vague, nonsensical, or irrational that it may not contain at least some personal, condensed meaning. In contrast to Wittgenstein, meaning in psychoanalysis is personal, dynamic, hierarchal, topographic, shifting. Whereas in Wittgenstein, and many analytic philosophers influenced by him, to say something meaningful is to confer a privileged, ontological status and to demonstrate something is meaningless is to deliver a powerful, ontological invalidation; much as the noted scientific philosopher, Karl Popper (Popper and Eccles 1977) uses the criterion of falsifiability to validate or invalidate scientific hypotheses. As analysts, we do not labor under the burden of having to *prove* meaning. For us meaning is ubiquitous; we have only to discover its manifestations and transformations. As analysts, we do not look at meaning as some logical essence or form (in the sense of Wittgenstein), which once found is static and fixed ("unassailable"); on the contrary, meaning for us can be transient, it can be forged before our eyes.

Language is important to psychoanalysis, but—allowing for

hermeneutic philosophers like Paul Ricoeur (1970) and metapsychological, linguistic revisionists like Roy Schafer (1976)—does not seem to carry the weight that it does for philosophers like Wittgenstein. Instead, psychoanalysis uses language as it does dreams, not as a fundamental stopping point but as a mediating, symbolic system (and therein tool) to be further deciphered, hopefully leading to even more fundamental, personal, relational meanings. The magical retrieval which David Pears (1969) so admired in Wittgenstein, was executed via the realigning of crossed metaphors and the unravelling of misapplied language pictures that had led to philosophical blind alleys. In psychoanalysis, if there is magical retrieval, it occurs because even the most nonsensical verbalizations and images (as for example in dreams) can—via interpretation—reveal personal meaning and intentionality. In this sense psychoanalysis, by accepting the language of the analysand in whatever shape it comes, uses language to *let in and restore* the world. It is a sharp contrast to Wittgenstein, whose paranoid style severely delimits the world, resulting in the previously mentioned loss of proportion and with it a loss of reality.

We might say, in their own ways, Wittgenstein and psychoanalysis use language to practice a different kind of linguistic abreaction: Wittgenstein through realigning crossed metaphors and unraveling misapplied language pictures—and thereby narrowing and purifying language—tries to lead the philosophical fly out of the bottle: while psychoanalysis, by hierarchically spreading the network of personal meaning to include every nonsensical, illogical, and irrational verbalization, by reconnecting through new associative pathways isolated affect to its proper idea, and by making even *silence* a vital part of communicative language (through interpreting it instead of banishing it as Wittgenstein does), tried to broaden, unrepress, and thereby restore the world.

Perhaps some of this is reflected in the respective writing styles of Wittgenstein and Freud. Both are acknowledged masters of German, but, paradoxically, Wittgenstein's style, presumably about nonworldly, abstract relationships, reveals more disturbance and inner conflict than Freud's, whose prose by comparison, though animated, introspective, and rich—in spite of the intensely charged world he is describing—is relatively self-contained and measured. This may be because the almost continuously charged nature of the pathological material he writes about is thereby somewhat cathartic and allows Freud to work through some of the anxiety necessarily provoked by the same material. By contrast, Wittgenstein, because of his need to bar the world and especially affect and deep personal meaning from his writing, is accordingly blocked and because of it has a greater need to release his powerful inner conflicts, which emerge in his famous, enigmatic style. As noted, never did a man expend so much feeling about so much abstraction.

Or perhaps it is simply that Wittgenstein's style, just because its content is so barren of emotion, *has* to be charged and dynamic, while Freud's style, just because the content is so charged and dynamic, must compensate by being more sober and self-contained. Whatever the cause, this much appears descriptively true: Wittgenstein's style with its darts and insights, its teasing, aphoristic slipperiness, and its tormented tone is more modern than Freud's. More modern because more self-conflictual and more ambivalent. The tension that exists between Wittgenstein and psychoanalysis exists between Wittgenstein's style and Wittgenstein's content. His style is passionate, dynamic, energetic, and filled with life. His content is the logically complete, inert world of the *Tractatus* or the language games and trivial-seeming ordinary language customs of the *Philosophical Investigations*. His style is unexpected, rich with surprise; his content is closed off, logically complete, gloomy, tautologous or alive in a trivial, behavioristic sense. By comparison, Freud's style, as dynamic and alive as Wittgenstein's, is at peace with its content. To us, it does not seem arbitrarily imposed on its subject matter as does Wittgenstein's. Instead, it seems to resonate with its subject matter and to grow naturally out it. Again, by contrast, Wittgenstein's restless tormented style—so at odds with the cold, formal world it describes—seems to spring, like Kafka's, from some great unknown inner depth. In terms of modern literature, Wittgenstein's style strikes us as more of what is called a *voice*. And we might conjecture that Freud—being able to express more of whatever personal conflicts he had in his writing—experienced a greater cathartic sense of release than Wittgenstein, *who was not able to achieve in his personal style linguistic abreaction; and so perhaps made linguistic abreaction—to let the fly out of the bottle—a consciously pursued, lifelong goal.*

To my knowledge, Freud and Wittgenstein never met. But Wittgenstein was aware of Freud ("Conversations on Freud," from *Wittgenstein Lectures and Conversations* 1972). It is no surprise that Wittgenstein was characteristically ambivalent toward Freud and highly critical. His remarks are instructive in how much of Freud they omit. Of course, it is to be expected that Wittgenstein will approach Freud on his own terms—linguistic analysis; but what is revealing is how thoroughly Wittgenstein chooses to ignore Freud on *his* terms. When Wittgenstein does touch on typical Freudian themes (the symbolism of dreams, the language of the unconscious), he seems to do so in an offhand, coolly appraising, almost ironically detached way. Noticeably missing is Wittgenstein's familiar, passionate engagement. One gets the strong impression that Wittgenstein wants nothing to do, wants to keep his distance very much, from the all too human, unmeasured world of psychoanalysis. His remarks may always be subtle, but Wittgenstein seems so out of sympathy with the spirit of psychoanalysis that his presence seems almost alien.

Although he consistently criticized it, Wittgenstein appears more at home in the world of science. As noted by Malcolm (1958) Wittgenstein's prodigious range of natural gifts extended from music, philosophy, and the arts, all the way to mechanical and aeronautical engineering, to mathematics and physics. Now it may be there is an analogy between Wittgenstein and the so-called reality crisis presently occurring in quantum mechanics (Herbert 1987); that is, that by reducing the physical world to a network of only formalized, abstract relationships there is a consequent loss of reality (even for physicists). Whether the world at bottom—the so-called deep reality—is really made up of only ordinary objects (the neorealist position of Einstein, Schrodinger, and others) or has no deep reality and is founded on probability outcomes of events (Heisenberg, Bohr) is a matter for particle physicists to decide. Yet psychologically it may be that the current, more orthodox physicist's view concerning reality (there is *no* deep reality, only probability outcomes of events) has as its price a consequent disconnection and sense of a loss of reality.

This sense of the loss of reality (induced in physicists as well as others) by the disconnected world of quantum mechanics reminds us of the fragmentation of the *Tractatus Logico-Philosophicus*. Though entirely different disciplines, modern linguistic analysis, founded in large measure by Wittgenstein, and modern quantum mechanics have in common that both reduce a rich world of objects (linguistic and physical) to abstract patterns, a minimal array of rules and relationships. There is a necessary loss of reality in both disciplines (Barrett 1979; Herbert 1985).

In contrast to both, psychoanalysis adopts a position—regarding the nature of the so-called deep reality—that in quantum reality terms (Herbert) would be called neorealism. This means that the ultimate reality psychoanalysis is describing is composed, if one looks far enough, of only ordinary objects, or rather, abstractions resembling ordinary objects. This, of course, follows from psychoanalysis' theoretical choice of stopping at instinct, near the border of psyche and soma thereby never giving itself a chance of getting to a subatomic, fundamental object that would not be considered ordinary by quantum reality standards or realistic (in the classical physicist's sense). While it may be objected that early psychoanalytic metapsychology seemed to abstract regions of the mind, it is also true that the abstractions are abstractions of what Herbert calls ordinary objects; here there are no probability waves and probability outcomes. The abstractions are abstractions of instinctual, affective, relational, neuronal, energetic entities—all ordinary objects. This is quite different from Wittgenstein whose world foundation (especially in the *Tractatus*), far from being composed of ordinary objects, is made up only of rule and linguistic extensions of pure logic. And further, if we are persuaded by Pribram and Gill (1976) then even the abstractions of Freud's metapsychology are, at bottom, transposed neurophysiological concepts (and therefore, according to Pribram, ordinary and testable).

This is only one more way of showing how psychoanalysis differs from Wittgenstein's linguistic analysis in that it uses language to restore the world. There is nothing that transpires in psychoanalysis no matter how inexact, blurred, irrational or disguised that may not be traced back to some personal ordinary object (instinctual, object relational)—and thereby made meaningful. In this sense, psychoanalysis uses language to restore the world in a way that linguistic philosophers like Wittgenstein do not.

It may be objected that psychoanalysis, in its effort to use language for more than logic and precision, moved too far beyond Wittgenstein and the logical positivists that followed him. It may be that the efforts of philosophers of science like Edelson (1984) and language purifiers like Roy Schafer (1976) are called for in order to bring psychoanalysis and analytic philosophers somewhat closer. But there is a difference between great systematizers like David Rapaport (1976) who need to pay exquisite attention to every nuance of psychoanalytic terminology in order to clarify theoretical concepts, and metapsychological revisionists like Roy Schafer (1976) who wish to revamp psychoanalysis on the basis of a streamlined language.

We suggest that the different uses of language by psychoanalysis and Wittgenstein are crucial and should not be overlooked. We characterize the language of psychoanalysis as *broad and open* to the extreme; it can accommodate the paranoid style of a Wittgenstein as well as every other neurotic style; it incorporates the language of dreams, the language of symbols, the language of the unconscious. By comparison, Wittgenstein's use of language, especially in the *Tractatus*—a work of first-rate philosophical genius—is extraordinarily *closed*. Finally, we suggest that it is this same versatility and openness of language in psychoanalysis, with so many linguistic threads running to the inner and outer world, that adds to its curative value. It is this ability through openness to restore the world, to always find meaning and personal centeredness, that, in the long run makes the use of language in psychoanalysis therapeutic.

In summary, we have taken the paranoid neurotic style, in the sense of David Shapiro (1965), and applied it to the full-blown philosophical genius of Wittgenstein. It is suggested that important aspects of his thought and style are thereby clarified. It is further suggested that the peculiar tension that exists between Wittgenstein and psychoanalysis arises from this same tension that exists *within* Wittgenstein between his neurotically restrictive paranoid style and the uncontrollable imaginative flow of his creative genius. Finally, the language of Wittgenstein—in spite of the profundity of its analysis—is characterized as essentially closed (despite valiant later efforts to "reverse" himself), while the language of psychoanalysis is characterized as exceptionally open—and therein therapeutic.

7
The Psychoanalyst: As True and False Self

So far, I have only touched on some of the personal (countertransferential) issues experienced in being a therapist working with young artists. They pertain, of course, not only to artists but to all patients and so important are they that they deserve at least an entire chapter to themselves.

One of Winnicott's seminal contributions to patient pathology was his conceptualization of the true and false self (1960). It will be my principal point that this conceptualization can as well be applied to the countertransferences of the analyst, the analytic situation itself, and even the analytic technique.

In his fundamental paper, "Ego Distortion in Terms of True and False Self" (1960), Winnicott has more to say about the false self than the true. He seems to see the true self more as the root and foundation (beginning in infancy with the tending of the good enough mother) of all subsequent healthy living and development. He likens the true self to the "spontaneous gesture" (p. 148). By contrast, Winnicott says of the false self, "This compliance, on the part of the infant, is the earliest stage of the false self.... The False Self has one positive and very important function ... to hide the True Self, which it does by compliance with environmental demands" (p. 147). He concludes with the crucial statement: *"Whereas, the True Self feels real, the existence of a False Self results in a feeling unreal or a sense of futility"* (p. 148).

Although in what follows, I draw mainly from psychoanalysis and my own experiences as a psychoanalytic psychotherapist (because that is what I know best), what is said can be applied as well to all dynamic relationship-based, and insight-oriented psychotherapies.

First, in order to show you what I mean by the idea of an analyst being a false self, I would like to present some personal encounters. Anyone who has ever attended one of the numerous therapy training institutes that presently prevail in Manhattan should be able to identify (if only partially) with them. While true (and, I believe, representative) they are not meant as horror stories, across-the-board caricatures, nor as isolated instances. Instead, they portray a type of false-self analyst who appears with enough regularity to be disturbing and comes in various roles, depicted here, respectively, as a young candidate, as a faculty supervisor, and as a famous analyst.

As a Candidate

The candidate is one of the golden boys of the institute I attended. He is tall, bearded, imposing, assured in word and gesture, armed with a Ph.D. from a prestigious university, and commands the respect of student, teacher, and supervisor alike. He is even rumored to be a secret favorite of the director. He likes me, and while I do not feel close to him, I admire his single-mindedness, his uncloudy sense of professional integrity, and his obvious high intelligence. I even forgive him his aggressive worship of Kohut, his penchant for preaching self psychology at a drop of a pin.

The time I speak of, what I most remember, occurs several years after the last seminar in which we both participated. I am happily surprised to bump into him at the office of a mutual friend and eagerly inquire as to the events of the intervening years. I mean this, socially; the response I am looking for is not a career progress report. But the candidate thinks otherwise, stiffens, and announces, "I'm a full-fledged self psychologist." He says this so coldly and condescendingly that I am taken aback, puzzled, hurt. I search my memory for something I may have done to trigger this, come up with nothing, while he continues, "I mean, look, if you're a physicist you don't waste time studying phlogiston." He cannot help now but note my welling, wounded indignation; pauses, adds boyishly and impishly, "At least that's my bias."—then, as I am about to respond, abruptly excuses himself to prepare for a patient's visit.

I tell this incident because it marks a revealing shift in my perspective of a colleague I have known for a decade. For ten years I have been observing him relate to colleagues, teachers, friends in a familiar pattern of formality, creation of a haughty barrier, condescension to the point of hurting, boyish reparation (upon seeing the hurt), then, speedy abandonment. Now, moments later, as I watch him smile, greet, and attend to a patient about to enter his office, I find myself straining to imagine what it would be like, from the patient's standpoint, to have an analytic experience with him. I wonder, where does the haughtiness go? Does it really dissolve before he gets into the office? Is it really left behind?

As a Faculty Supervisor

Her face is gaunt and weather-beaten; she is smart as a whip, brooks no nonsense, and treats her supervisees with an imperiousness she does not attempt to hide. Things go her way or they do not go at all. Her method of supervision is cold, businesslike, domineering: she seems more focused on showcasing the talents she presumes she has than on listening to or helping the supervisee. How she became a tenured faculty supervisor is a mystery, but it is a fact she became one.

The time I speak of is twelve years ago and my friend, fledgling colleague—to become one of the best analysts I know—is in a state of analytic crisis. He is struggling with his first assigned case with this same woman: he is shocked now to discover his supervisor—without a single word of discussion—has gone behind his back straight to the director and requested that all future patient referrals be canceled. My friend's career as a budding analyst is on the line. He does not know what to do. He knows his supervisor, clearly, has violated an unspoken code of conduct. He also knows she has the power to get away with it. And we both know, to be open and approach her with the truth of his findings, as he is required to do, would be asking for even more trouble, because the truth would have to be on the order of, "I feel it was despicable of you to go behind my back instead of dealing with me face to face and the fact your only interest in me seems to be in using me to inflate your power as a supervisor is just about ruining what little confidence I have left as a novice therapist."

It is not hard to figure out what, most likely, she would do: listen in silent rage and then do her best to punish my friend under the shield of confronting his pathological resistances. So I come up with, I get, what feels like a daring idea, even a revolutionary idea, if you consider the context and strictures of the institute I attend (i.e., you never dream of challenging the supervisor assigned to you). Don't approach her with the truth—change supervisors! Invent an excuse—mandatory job change, for instance, necessitating new scheduling of free hours; express due regrets, and move on (to freedom).

I tell this because it marks a loss of innocence: the beginning of a certain (unfortunately necessary) gamesmanship that is imposed on one when dealing with the pathological types one must occasionally encounter in positions of genuine power.

As a Famous Analyst

This is seven years ago in a packed, Upper East Side auditorium. The famous analyst, a self-styled apostle of Robert Langs, who considers himself even more purist in his handling of the frame than the master himself, is presenting. His method of presentation is to bring two subordinate presenters along and then publicly supervise them. The demonstration, as I recall, begins with a temporary malfunctioning of the microphone, but the famous analyst waves away the repairman's attempt to adjust the microphone, and even the microphone itself. He doesn't need one; and indeed for six hours, minus a lunch break, his booming voice uninterruptedly fills the hushed auditorium.

But it is not his platform delivery, remarkable though it is, that I find so fascinating. It is the style of his interacting, or rather noninteracting, with his two subordinate presenters (a man and a woman, both dignified, utterly serious, professional therapists). He treats them not as people but as simple vehicles or vessels through which to implement what he obviously believes is a godlike technique. He therefore does not feel obligated to listen to more than a sentence or two before immediately interrupting ("You can sit down"), taking over, and grandiosely pontificating, amazingly, sometimes for stretches up to an hour.

A friend, who is sitting and suffering with me, afterward puts all of this in perspective for me when she says, "I have no idea, of course, what it must be like to be in therapy with him, but if the insensitivity he showed (consistently) to his presenters is any indication, I have to wonder." I tell this because it is another revelation, the first time I realize (though, of course, I cannot prove it) that even a famous therapist—far from being the great clinician he proclaims himself to be—could, in actuality, be a poor one.

You may say that such examples of the analyst as a false self—seriously dissociated from any contact with a real, alive, spontaneous, creative, true self (in the Winnicottian sense)—may occur: but that they will not occur in a really good institute. Isn't it the very job of an institute to weed out the insufferable candidates? Yet the answer is, even the best institutes regularly fail. We all know impossible people—while they may not be iatrogenic to their patients, neither are they therapeutic—who not only get through the face to face evaluations of institutes with flying colors, but keep rising to positions of power and prominence. How does this happen? Well, therapists have their game faces, too. They know the right moves. Not an insignificant part of their craft and expertise in human relations is an awareness of just what is expected of them in a multitude of roles and social interactions.

By trying to look at analysts this way, from a Winnicottian perspective, as true and false selves, it is not meant to imply that every time we encounter a colleague or teacher, we should expect an uplifting, growth-enhancing, magical experience. It does not mean, that in order to be in the presence of what we mean by a true self, not a false self analyst, we should be added to at least once in every five-minute encounter.

It does mean, though, that we should not feel less, restricted in ourselves, feel bad, trifled with, demeaned, alienated, put in our place; and that if we do, and if we can trust our instincts that it was not an accident, or a bad day, but the person involved was really doing something interactively to our particular vulnerabilities, then that can be a warning signal. A signal more reliable than, for example, sitting and comfortably attending knowledgeable lectures on the history of technique which ought to bespeak a respected, accomplished, and seasoned clinician.

How can a person who has a talent for somehow bringing out the worst in ourselves and others, and for helping us to feel not good about ourselves, change hats and be the same person (as analyst) who can sustain patients for years, at the most tender, raw and vulnerable recesses of their psyches? The answer, I think, is obvious enough to fall in the emperor-has-no-clothes category. They can't. To the degree they are seriously dissociated from their own real, true, alive, spontaneous, and creative selves, do they fail their patients. And rather than pass on, and facilitate, a higher, richer, and more integrated level of intimacy, it is more likely they bequeath to their patients, in disguised form, their own defensive (false self) strategies for living.

Roy Schafer has written beautifully of what he terms in the analyst a second self (1983), a kind of higher, analytic ego-ideal. He likens it to the writer's authorial self, someone who can achieve magnificent heights of nobility while writing ("write like an angel," p. 44) yet, who can often be "above average in their everyday misery, cruelty, greed, egocentricity, snobbery, self-destructiveness and sociopathy" (p. 44). The analogy does not exactly hold. The writer does not relate directly to his intended audience, but only through the disembodied, symbolic intermediary of his art. By contrast, the analyst has no proxy. He relates directly with his voice, his gesture, his body language, his whole living presence.

It is the position taken here that if the analyst is one of Schafer's magnificent, authorial selves, who, in reality, is clearly "above average in everyday misery, cruelty, greed, egocentricity, snobbery, self-destructiveness and sociopathy," then sooner or later it will show. The patient will figure it out and no higher second self available is going to save him or her. A more faithful analogy to the authorial self than Schafer's second self might be the authorial analyst, i.e., the fictive analyst in *I Never Promised You a Rose Garden* (1964), supposedly Frieda Fromm Reichman, the personal favorite of my youth. I don't know how I would have reacted had I encountered her analytically. I might have loved her, or hated her, or more probably, a mixture of both.

This brings us to a consideration of the analytic situation itself, in terms of Winnicott's formulation of a true and false self.

In our view it is a crucial fact that seen in this light, in certain intrinsic, inescapable features, *the analytic situation, itself, does not feel real—it feels false.*

This is meant as a description, not a critique, because the belief here is that the analytic situation is the way it is, because it has to be that way to ensure its objectivity and frame. If so, then what are the intrinsic, inescapable features contributing to its perceived interpersonal falseness?

Because of its structured, artificial setup, its analytic rules of behavior, and tight frame, the analytic situation will necessarily always lack a certain fluid, spontaneous, open-ended creativity that any other (nonrule-governed) dynamic, whole, human relationship can have. It is in this sense, that the analytic relationship can never, by its constituent nature and frame, be experienced as a whole relationship, but always as a part or piece of a human relationship. That is why it does not feel real.

It would be one thing if the analytic relationship presented itself as only a highly formalized part, however significant, of a genuine human relationship. But it also asks itself to be viewed as potentially one of the most intimate, meaningful, psychic journeys imaginable, and therein lies the paradox. A highly formalized, mysterious, rule-governed analyst, on the one hand, whose behavior—no matter how idealistically invested in his role, falls under the category of professionally working for a profit—and, on the other hand, the analysand, generally emotionally vulnerable, unstable, looking for a psychic bond that may be disturbing, thrilling, a rescue, a cure, a growth experience, a higher form of intimate relating, a stalemate, a puzzlement.

The two don't go together. They never have. Double bind theorists like Haley (1968) are not just smart-aleck gadflies who delight in giving us a hard time: they really have put their finger on something. Of course, they go much too far, they take the black box view of the psyche, say everything is caused by the environmental double bind, and arrive at the simplistic therapeutic strategy: let's manipulate the manipulator (double bind)! By contrast, analysts, historically, have tended to protect the analytic situation by denying the existence or potency of the double bind paradox: even interpersonal analysts such as the Sullivanians who tend to see the analytic situation as a participant, constructivist field generally do not talk about or perceive deficits, per se, in the interpersonal field of the analytic situation itself.

For these reasons, the analytic situation scarcely ever sits entirely right with the patient. This will be true even for patients who have had good analyses, good therapeutic alliances, and the true benefits of analysis demonstrated to them (internally and externally) numerous times. It can also be true for analytic candidates, practitioners, even teachers in the field. It takes years of training and experience for a candidate to begin to feel comfortable in the analytic role. Some analysts never do. This may be why even presumably healthy people who are undergoing a didactic analysis manifest their share of transferential reactions and are never resistance-free.

Seen in this way, there may be an area of transference analysis that has been neglected. Transference may not just be the outcome of regressive illness or reaction to objects (internal, external). It may in addition be a normal (as well as transferential) outcome: an attempt at reparation to make a relationship (analytic situation) that does not sit right, feel whole, or real—into one more whole and more real. If this is so, patients may not only be projecting and manifesting derivatives of their intrapsychic sense of conflict and fragmentation. They may also be projecting and manifesting a sense of interpersonal fragmentation, peculiar to the analytic situation, that is *real* (not transferentially distorted). The splits patients are struggling to resist, defend themselves against, or to heal *may also include splits in the analytic relationship.*

Perhaps because it can be a narcissistic injury to their personal humanism, analysts tend to deny or minimize the pain that is caused by the analytic relationship itself and see it instead as intrapsychic resistance. Unlike physicians who can reasonably attempt to quantitatively justify the pain contained in their treatment, through a cost versus benefits analysis, analysts can never be sure the pain they are causing will ever be justified. What they need is the stamina Roy Schafer talks about (1983, p. 48), the ability to see the payoff, and to wait for the payoff that is ahead. For all of these reasons, analysts do not spend enough time analyzing the distortions and splits implicit in the analytic situation, and spend too much time analyzing patient distortions within the analytic situation.

We do not mean it pejoratively when we say there is a deficit, a stiltedness, deprivation, and impoverishment implicit in the analytic situation and analytic relationship that is real (not transferential). We choose to see it as a realistic, descriptive confrontation of an undeniable fact. To make a trade-off, to try to breathe in more fluidity and dynamic spontaneity by opening up the frame, would ruin the objectivity that is central to the analytic enterprise. We know that when psychoanalytic psychotherapy works (admitting this is not always the case), there is an enrichment in living that far transcends that which preceded it—and which, by the way, is our proof, the only real proof we will ever get, of the value of our work.

The paradox, the double bind of psychoanalysis is that it begins with a shrinkage, a lessening, a deprivation, in terms of human relating, and finishes with a flourish, a true enrichment. But this in no way denies or repudiates the real deprivation as perceived by the patient. The ways we have of analytically relating to our patients *are* painful and the perceived pain is not transferential. On the other hand, it is probable that it is easier for patients to accept this than for us, because this fact can always feed their negative transference.

If this is so, there might be a concept of the *real resistance* (as in real relationship versus transferential relationship) wherein it is understood that there is a certain (and necessary) artificiality, restrictedness, and unreality implicit in the analytic situation which the patient will eventually perceive and (appropriately) resist. In this sense, at least some of what is usually called the patient's resistance will be an attempt to either defend itself or break through the false and unreal-seeming analytic situation per se, in an effort to find and talk to the suspected hidden true self of the analyst. I think this is why we sometimes have the impression in our practice that the technique we are using, the role we are assuming, is not so much a facilitator as a barrier to the patient. If only we could strip it away (which we know we can't) perhaps the patient might really say what he or she wants to say.

In another realm, this may explain why so much of our psychiatric, psychoanalytic literature comes off as stale, mechanical, and terminologically dreary. It is not just that there may be an insufficiency of enlivening, able writers among us who can add art and sparkle to our craft. It may also be that much of what we do *is* dreary, stale, mechanical, and terminological, and in part is forced upon us by the deficits of the analytic situation.

By contrast, the writings of R. D. Laing and Harold Searles, though occasionally they may baffle us with their quaintness, do not bore us. Their imaginative brilliance aside, this can be because each of them seems freely to share or hint at deep personal problems and to be comfortable with their personal deficits. They do not present themselves as experts holding tightly to the reins of a near perfect technique. They emerge more as poets of suffering rather than neat, clinical dissectors of the psyche: analysts who themselves are sometimes baffled, sometimes faltering; who have breakthroughs, but who also stumble. Because they seem to move so freely and fluidly through their individual analytic space they strike us, and others, as poignantly, charmingly real.

The Flight from Unreality

There is a historical element to be considered. If the analytic situation, as suggested, implies or fosters a paradoxical unreality, a certain falseness, this may help explain some of the more radical therapies that have been spinoffs (in a sense) of psychoanalysis. It may be that certain radical departures from classical psychoanalytic technique—for example, gestalt and psychodrama—have been motivated, in part, by what was believed to be a necessary and invigorating *flight from the unreality of the analytic situation.* It may be that some of the excesses (from our eyes) of gestalt and psychodrama technique are none other than a wild, exuberant attempt to pump more life, more spontaneity, and more realness into what is perceived as a mechanical, anesthetic, straitjacketed, analytic technique. Yet, there is a catch here: gestalt and psychodrama therapies, in their eagerness to cram unfettered, impulsive spontaneity into their repertoire of techniques, become hoist on their own petard, (in this case double bind).

This is because the issues of unreality, from which gestalt and psychodrama technique wish to separate themselves, can in turn become acute in techniques that came to be based on *caricatures* of a human relationship. Gestalt therapy, with its use of the hot seat, its frank encouragement of an array of exhibitionistic forms of expression in patients, can be so bizarrely unreal that any resemblance to a human relationship ceases to exist. Behavior becomes broken apart and spoken of in terms of a discrete series of exercises and techniques, while psychodrama, well before a relationship can begin, allows reality to be grandly swept away before a series of imaginary personae.

This is not to deny powerful affects often emerge. They do, but it may be one reason gestalt and psychodrama therapies are populated with so many powerful, theatrical therapists is that only such a therapist is capable of sweeping away the feeling of unreality that is ironically induced by their bizarre attempts to achieve what they think is the truly real. Therefore, gestalt and psychodrama therapists, while they may be deeply connected to their patients, can also have a relationship that in some ways mirrors the bond between actor and audience. Some of their therapeutic skill may lie in their ability to create an illusion of reality (the way an actor does); and it may be a reason so often there is little lasting effect to encounter experiences and encounter therapies in general, is that there can also be little more relationship between therapist and patient than between actor and audience.

One last word on the eclectic therapist. In my experience I have met few if any genuine eclectic therapists, but I have met many who have called themselves that. This may not be so much the confident claim of competence in a variety of techniques as a *defense* against being considered rigid, artificial, unreal—as though the flexibility and breath of life promised in being called eclectic might somehow cancel out the prospective patient's imagined dread of being asphyxiated in a single technique. This denies the basic fact there is enough space in the major techniques—Freudian, Sullivanian, Jungian, self psychology—to absorb for the entirety of one's life even the most gifted of therapists, without having to add, "I may be this, but I am also that and that."

Although what we have said so far has been directed primarily to analysts and the analytic situation, it can also apply, in varying measures, to all dynamic psychotherapies: whenever there is that strange, unsettling, incongruous admixture of role-governed, rule-bound, fee-oriented, professional behavior enjoined to a firm expectation of continuously candid, self-exploration and intimate psychic bonding. In this regard, we have spoken—from a Winnicottian perspective—of a false self: first as pertaining to the countertransferences of the analyst, then as pertaining to the analytic situation itself. But what of a false technique?

There will be as many false techniques as there are false analytic selves, but a common one will center on a belief in a code of conduct for the therapist so protected that it is held to be almost universally true. To show the difficulty with this (although I personally believe the ethical constraints implicit in being a good psychotherapist can never be overestimated) I have tried to come up with a rule of behavior for analysts and psychotherapists, so self-evidently true that it can guarantee, in advance, near complete agreement. The first choice is the obvious choice: never have sex with your patients. This can be discarded almost immediately because increasingly the rule is being challenged, not only by radical therapists, but, unfortunately, by pathological therapists.

So, in the search for a rule of conduct for analysts that will be universally accepted, we have to move to the other pole of behavior: aggression. Note that already a pattern is emerging: in order to have any hope of finding a rule of conduct that will gain general, or near general approval, we must forsake all subtlety and nuance and concentrate on the gross extremities of behavior. I do this and arrive at the following rule of behavior for analysts, guaranteed to win universal acceptance: no matter how provoked you may feel yourself to be, never become physically aggressive with your patients. No one, of course, has ever contested this. So here we have a self-evident, universally agreed-upon rule of conduct for analysts.

But there's a catch. So far we have been talking only in the ethereal, abstract code of conduct realm. What happens if we take our hypothetical universal rule and put it into real life, where the screw always gets turned, where it is less easy, and where universally self-evident rules of conduct are yet to be found? Suppose, for example, while I know of no one who has ever advocated getting physically aggressive with our patients, we slightly change the question and ask, "Are we ever, and if so to what extent, entitled as analysts to defend ourselves, if physically assaulted by our patients?" (We are asking the *same question,* but by altering the temporal sequence and context—from aggressor to defender—the mental picture radically changes from the psychotic one of us rising from our chair to physically abuse our patients to the sane one of our being forced to defend ourselves against a patient who is psychotic.)

Now if the answer is yes, as some analysts will surely reply, a new question immediately presents itself. Is there a prescribed way (a therapeutic, textbook way) to defend ourselves? Do we passively ward off and neutralize intended blows, as we sometimes ward off and neutralize intended psychic battering, and thereby provide a corrective experience of what a nonretaliatory, benign object would do?

Whatever the answer, there is an obvious, important, physical question: who is bigger or stronger than whom?—that also demands our attention. Major countertransferential issues can arise depending on how we perceive the assault: is it only a pitiful, childlike attempt to shake out of a yearned-for parent figure more needed love and attention, or is it a full-blooded, sociopathic onslaught with a serious intent to maim? Or are these questions irrelevant, because once physical violence enters the picture, all bets are off, the analyst–patient contract is irrevocably broken (along, perhaps, with our narcissistic pride), and we are free to defend ourselves as vigorously and aggressively as is required?

Obviously, there will be as many and as varying responses to our hypothetical question as there are analysts. The fact that such patient assaults are rare in private practice (none has occurred to me or to anyone I know) in no way resolves the theoretical issue that is being raised. If only because such assaults do in fact occur in the more seriously disturbed, psychotic population of hospitalized patients, which is why attendants are often posted by the door for therapy sessions with patients judged potentially violent. The point is once you take even the most seemingly universal, self-evident rule of conduct (never become physically aggressive with patients) out of the vacuum of nonliving, abstract discussion, that is, once you bring it to life, variables that you did not think of will always arise.

Take one more example. It is hard to imagine anyone disagreeing with the beautiful maxim—the physician (analyst) should never be iatrogenic (bring harm to the patient). Yet, once we take it out of the abstract and into the treatment situation, an immediate dilemma arises. Since analytic therapy, to some degree, inasmuch as it is not primarily based on immediate alleviation of symptoms, is dependent on the emergence and toleration of shifting degrees of discomfort, tension, anxiety, and psychic stress, the question arises: at what point, when we begin to suspect or know that no therapeutic gain is in sight for the patient in manifest stress, do we try to intervene and modulate that useless anxiety? To that point, that we are comfortable or uncomfortable with what we deem useless and disabling anxiety, will we be considered supportive or unsupportive, unduly strict, or appropriately neutral (depending on the observer's viewpoint).

If your position is any amount of anxiety is justified and does not need intervention, you do not thereby sidestep the dilemma, because then you are merely adopting the most extreme position possible on the subject, and although you may be right, there is a very good chance you are wrong—and if you are wrong, then you are being iatrogenic (whether you mean to be or not) and you have to take responsibility for it.

What a false technique does, according to the view we are presenting here, is to attach itself to such a principle and hold onto it as a *substitute for a therapeutic self*. It then searches the reality of the clinical situation for the best match it can find; subsequently judging the success or failure of the technique by the accuracy and closeness of the fit.

We can summarize this by saying that a false self technique, or false technique, emerges whenever there is an attempt to somehow quantify the interaction of a supposed principle of behavior with a live clinical situation. Such false self technique arises when there is an attempt to predict behavior, when there is a belief that there is a correct, sanitized code of behavior that can be projected into the future—like a predictive hypothesis—and experimentally (i.e., in the clinical here and now) confirmed or falsified (Langs 1988). By contrast, the good analyst's technique does not *precede* treatment, but imaginatively evolves and is validated in the course of treatment. Finally, the most commonly used defense (because it is easiest) of the false self of the analyst is the employment of a sterile, false technique: even more than neutrality, it can provide a defensive haven for countertransferences, especially false self countertransferences in which the analyst, as has been noted, is heavily invested in being or appearing radically other than he or she is.

By talking about the false self techniques, it is not meant to imply there is anything wrong with our principles: neutrality, empathy, objectivity, the frame, the interpretive stance. They have stood the test of time, no matter how hotly they are debated, because they are the best we have. But they are located within. They are not tried and true recipes in the cookbook of correct therapeutic behavior. Although they have been here much of the century, they are in no sense finished rules waiting to be copied. Rather, are they waiting to be transformed, to be born even (and in no sense are alive and operative until so done). In order to apply any of these principles beneficially in the clinical here and now there are perhaps hundreds of variables and thousands of permutations to be taken into account that have scarcely been touched upon in the literature. It takes a rich, cohesive sense of self, a fine-tuned clinical sensibility, unique timing, and above all, empathic imagination and artistry to do it. Not surprisingly, it doesn't happen often. A good analyst is almost as rare as a good artist.

We have saved the concept of analyst as true self for last, as Winnicott did. It is easy to say the good analyst must bring his true self to the analytic situation. But what are the attributes of the true self that will especially pertain to the good analyst? Every analyst will have his own list, but here is mine.

1. *Therapeutic personality (which includes warmth).* First of all, it is obvious that someone can be their creative, spontaneous, alive, true self and still be nasty, (if that is part of their true self). So the true self must be therapeutic. And now we can immediately define what we mean by a therapeutic personality. *A therapeutic personality is a true self whose presence is therapeutic.*

2. *Empathic imagination.* You can be a good doctor without imagination. You can be a good physicist without imagination. But you can't be a good therapist without imagination. It takes imagination to leap nimbly from self to self and then back again. Kohut's (1978) important concept of introspective empathy and the empathic stance seems to take for granted the critical factor of imagination. Empathic is always empathic imagination. To be always anxiously attending to the needs of a narcissistic or depressed mother does not in itself make for empathy, it can also make for being excessively attentive to the needs of the other. To turn it into true empathy, to be able to objectively see and understand the other's world through the other's eyes, requires the kind of imaginative leap made, for example, by the writer, who, with only limited experience and observation of another's existence, can sometimes, vividly, reconstitute a chunk of a life. That is why true empathy is more than a trait on a personality profile. It is a gift of imagination.

3. *Kindness.* It is so taken for granted that the quality of kindness is an important ingredient in therapeutic, human relating that it is never spoken about. We have to go outside analytic

literature to find a prominent author who takes kindness seriously as a topic worth writing about—all the way to Kurt Vonnegut (1982). Yet it is a sad fact that there are people who habitually frequent training institutes who are not kind. They may not be iatrogenic or abrasive, but neither do they possess any manifest degree of kindness that seems appropriate to the special poignancy that each patient in his or her unique way brings to the treatment: and sometimes is the *only* sensitive intervention. Patients, of course, will stick it out for years with an unkind therapist—if only because it recreates a familiar scenario between themselves and an indifferent parent—but one wonders, without the benefit of a benign, therapeutic introject, how much genuine progress can really be made.

4. *Clinical sensibility and artistry.* This is not to deny a place for competent, though uninspired therapy. A therapist with a basic sense of self, some sensitivity, and a certain good fellowship—but no special breadth of clinical sensibility or gift of artistry—can definitely carry a patient (someone who is suffering and ready to make a connection) farther than he or she was before entering treatment. But not much farther.

Because of this (and many other traits) good training institutes are aware that what the candidate brings to the institute is more important than what the institute brings to the candidate. But institutes do not talk about what cannot be taught (naturally). They only talk about what can be taught. It is natural that a false equation gets set up in the minds of trainees: technique = that which is taught; and that which is not taught is not technique. On the contrary, *the technique that cannot be taught, is more important than the technique that can be taught.* This does not mean to challenge the place of good training and a good institute, which is invaluable. A candidate can no more make himself or herself into a true analyst than a patient can execute a legitimate self-cure. It does mean that Langs's frame, no matter how expertly administered, unless it, in *turn, is itself framed or held in the therapeutic (whatever those qualities may be) true self of a good analyst will have little or no impact on a patient.*

The Good Enough Analyst

In his paper on the true and false self, Winnicott spoke of the "good enough mother" (p. 145). According to the view being presented here, we can amend this to the *good enough analyst*.

The good enough analyst is comfortable with mistakes since he is not administering a godlike technique, and trusts the mistakes will not be iatrogenic. The good enough analyst knows that the relationship with the patient does not cease to exist unless some activity, intervention, or technique is being performed like some external procedure upon the patient. The good enough analyst knows that the relationship with the patient—especially if there is history and a good therapeutic alliance—will always *precede* the technique of the analyst (what is done).

Concerning the analytic relationship and the analytic situation, the good enough analyst will recognize and admit (at some level, I believe) its problematical, existential nature; senses that there is something forever incomplete, not whole, always denying, inherently contradictory, paradoxical, and incongruent and (to these degrees) unreal-feeling about the analytic situation; but also knows this does not mean that the *analyst as person* cannot be whole. And this is what the good enough analyst does: *holds* the human deficits and paradoxical splits of the analytic situation and heals them as well as possible *exactly* as he holds the deficits and splits *within* the patient. In this regard the good enough analyst knows that the best answer to the patient's frequent charge of falseness and unreality of the analytic situation is not more and better technique, not simply a passing-the-buck analysis of the patient's resistances. It is a genuine, therapeutic true self of the analyst that can contain and make more whole (therefore more bearable) the splits in the analytic situation.

For their part, patients have a job to do, too. We tend *to forget patients have to learn technique also and it is as difficult for them to learn as it is for us.* The technique they have to learn, of course, is not the technique of treatment issues. They have to learn that this strange silence is not meanness or withholding; that this maddening neutrality is not deadness nor hollowness; that this person who volunteers almost nothing personal about himself or herself is not hiding or afraid. In short, they must come to understand that technique is an aspect of a person, to relate to technique that way, and to trust it, if they can. They have to learn that the technique they first meet embedded in a person is somehow part of a long, therapeutic process, and part of a whole, therapeutic person, that may somehow benefit them.

To summarize: no new rules or changes in the analytic situation are being proposed. However, by applying Winnicott's ideas of a true and false self first to the countertransferences of the analyst, then to the analytic situation, and finally to the analytic technique, it is suggested both an interesting and original way of looking at some of the dynamic processes involved may be gained.

8
The Double Bind in Psychoanalysis

factors, while certainly not a third force in psychoanalysis—is nevertheless *real*. It is not only real but it may be seen as a powerful social stimulant permeating the analytic situation that has been largely overlooked.

Gregory Bateson (1956) conceived of the double bind as a kind of poignant, metacommunicational trap. A child is caught in a family nexus of multilevel, conflicting messages. Whichever way he turns, whatever is said or done, whatever is not said and not done, there is punishment, pain, puzzlement. The position is *untenable*, yet the position is hardened by a covert, second level parental message forbidding the child to leave the interpersonal field. Finally, a third, hidden parental injunction (which secures the trap) warns, "Do not talk about this."

Gregory Bateson (1956), Don Jackson (1956), Jay Haley (1958), R. D. Laing (1961), and a generation of family systems therapists decided to defy that frightening parental injunction. They would not only talk about the double bind, they would use and manipulate it. They would "sharpen the paradox" (Jackson and Haley, 1963, p. 125) in the hope of achieving faster relief and briefer psychotherapy. Perhaps by placing patients and their symptoms in a *new* (therapeutic) paradox, they could thereby take control of the very nature of the relationship, including paradoxical effects. Perhaps they could *force* change (behavioristically) without, necessarily, relying upon insight.

Regarding such techniques, as analysts we have no choice but to think there is more to therapy than issues of power and control. There is also an intricate affective and cognitive process between stimulus and response; and between therapist and patient (no matter how manipulative or directive the therapeutic strategy is), there is always a unique hierarchy of personal meanings that must be respected.

Nevertheless, as already mentioned, we differ from many analysts in that we think the double bind is both important and operative. Yet, we differ even more sharply from double bind theorists whose primary therapeutic, strategic goal—by posing a new, therapeutic paradox—is to unravel a suspected pathological, familial, metacommunicational bottleneck. By contrast, we see the

I began this book by describing some of the dou[ble binds en]countered by the artist in his relationship to his art, [...] and, especially (from our point of view), to his ther[apist. Over the] years, I gradually became aware that these double [binds applied] not only to the nonartistic patient but to the therap[ist and to the] therapeutic situation as well. And, therefore, before [concluding, I] feel obliged to briefly depict this overview of what [I believe is the] more general significance of the double bind in p[sychotherapy,] presented as in the previous chapter from the pers[pective I know] best—that is, from psychoanalysis and my own e[xperience as a] psychoanalytic psychotherapist.

Formally articulated by Gregory Bateson (19[56) and enthu]siastically incorporated into family systems theor[y (e.g.,] Haley 1963), the double bind has been largely r[elegated to the] status of fashionable, theoretical gadfly by analysts [...] In opposition to this I want to show that the doub[le bind is] not comparable in importance to the intrapsychic [...]

201

double bind, especially the analytic double bind, as essentially not one of paradoxical, mixed messages and conflicting levels of communication. Instead, we see it as arising *from a conflict of incompatible levels of intimacy: specifically, the (unspoken of) conflict between technique and intimacy.*

The central double bind, inasmuch as the analytic situation is concerned, is that the patient is put into *the role (or expectation) of nonreciprocal intimacy with a professional stranger.* The central double bind, as far as the analyst is concerned (in our view), is that—in a dyadic setting evocative of profound intimacy—he is constrained *to behave in a manner largely dictated by an impersonal, professional technique (regardless of how empathically that technique may be manifested).*

From the patients' viewpoint as analysands, we are asked on the one hand to slowly, regressively, sink to the deepest dependency, the most childlike transferential love (or hate); and then to organize ourselves and pay for it. We are asked to put two things together that in our culture are essentially antithetical and almost never go well together. The two things are structured, rule-defined, fee-oriented, nonreciprocal behavior with a firm request for the most candid, intimate, sustained self-disclosure and psychic bonding generally conceived.

There does not seem to be a relationship-analogue in our culture to help prepare the patient for the analytic situation. Role theory, with its emphasis on contextually appropriate and contextually governed behavior does not apply because the implied analogy to the physician to whom we carefully surrender a part of our bodies does not apply. There is a major difference between surrendering a part of our bodies to a physician, and what can seem the *whole* of our psyches to an analyst. When it is the precious autonomy of our self that we are being asked to share (and thereby perhaps lose) our interpersonal expectation, accordingly, can radically rise. And the fact that the analyst we meet—by the nature of his or her role— can easily seem the most guarded, mysterious person one has ever encountered only deepens the paradox and the double bind.

It is ironic that the two cultural roles that are perhaps closest as analogues to the analytic situation are parent/child and penitent/confessor or disciple/guru. Both are institutionalized forms of helplessness from which the patient is often presumably trying to escape (another double bind). The crucial difference, of course, is that the parent *is* the parent and the father confessor or guru *is* the institutionalized religious link to a transcendental, supposedly higher Being or way of being. In other words, even though these roles may certainly contain their special double binds, there is nevertheless considerable cultural justification and encouragement to bear up to and endure such double binds.

Nowhere near the same cultural sanctions pertain to the analyst, analysand, and analytic situation. The analyst is *not* a religious link to a higher power, to a higher way of being, and a higher knowledge (obvious though this may be, it is still sometimes surprisingly disregarded). You may counter that the role of analyst of course is sanctioned in our culture—if only in our pop culture and, (unfortunately) in an increasingly negative way.

But that is the point. Outside the special pleading of analytic and psychotherapeutic indoctrination, there is really almost nothing within our basic culture that speaks for the analysand's subordination of his psyche to a painful transferential regression that can often seem to be a dangerous helplessness. Far more difficult is it to subordinate the psyche to an analyst who is not only the most mysterious important person he may ever meet but who (confusingly) is neither a parent, priest, nor guru. By contrast, there is plenty in our culture that sanctions, in countless ways, the psychological and biological helplessness of the role of child and the role of religious penitent or disciple.

The Analyst's Dilemma

It is not only the patient who experiences and is caught up in the paradoxical effects of the psychoanalytic double bind. As analysts we are subject to certain ambiguities and perplexing open-ended questions which, no doubt, will be answered differently by each of us. Yet all of them may be seen to reflect, in some degree, an underlying double bind. For example, there is the question regarding our identity. Are we essentially objective professionals (with requisite warmth) who use our capacity for human relating basically as a tool to help? Or are we essentially committed, caring people who instead use our professional objectivity basically as a tool to help? Analysts who are especially unresolved in this may wear both hats but at different times. The double bind inherent in the analytic situation may allow them to switch, according to their countertransferential needs, from being intimate, caring, and empathic to being objective, professional, and ever vigilant of the frame.

Another question: To what extent and how do we deal with what might be called the "double standard of truthfulness" implied in the analytic situation? We refer to the fact that as analysts we have access to two distinct languages: one that we speak to patients, highly censored and on our own terms; and one that we speak to colleagues, out of earshot of our patients, which is immeasurably franker, freer, and less censored. We cannot help but note the discrepancy for patients for whom we always encourage but one language (which holds almost nothing back and is as close as possible to the ultimate in self-disclosure).

How do we sort out the professional need to evaluate time as money from the corresponding (patient's) need for us to be fully and humanly present in the here and now; and, therefore, to a certain extent, to be empathically *blinded* to time? There is no simple answer to this. Analysts especially unclear on this issue may experience the shadow of the clock—which can notoriously come into play whenever there is an overrun ("Your time is up")—as continuously hovering over the session, like a meter running. The allusion to therapists, one sometimes hears, as being almost prostitutes of relating—"You're the only one who listens to me, but I'm paying you"—is not just hostility. It is also rooted in the fact that there is no analogue in our culture for selling our relating. The artist who has to set a price tag on his art may be the closest we can come. Yet the artist can rely upon a somewhat natural temporal division between the process of his art and the subsequent marketing of his art and use that to separate them.

The double bind is much greater for the therapist who cannot take refuge in any such clean division (much as he and his patient might try their best to isolate the economics of therapy from the process and purpose of therapy). By contrast, the therapist works by the hour, charges by the hour, and can easily be perceived as doing a kind of glorified, humane, piecework. There is a sense, economically speaking, that therapists are ruled by the clock. This sobering truth, if it needs any reinforcement, is reflected in our income tax form. We do estimated taxes. We are listed as self-employed businessmen and businesswomen.

It is logical, then, to ask what is our business? If we are a business, what is our product? Are we delivering the product we deliver in our economic pursuit of an attractive profit? Or, is it the other way around? Are we really essentially unmaterialistic (though we may appreciate and enjoy the benefits of being financially comfortable)? Are we, instead, just realists who have made a decision to try and earn a living doing the thing we most love, and therefore accept that there is an unavoidable business aspect to what we do? Few therapists are sufficiently clear on this point. They should not be since the culture they live in isn't. Finally, there is the confusing question: What percentage of our interest in a given session is interest in the patient, and what percentage of our interest is interest in earning the fee for that session?

An Artificial Human Laboratory

We suggest an analogy, admittedly crude, to help explain how the analytic double bind we are postulating may have arisen. Conceive of the analytic situation as an artificial, human laboratory and compare it with a scientific laboratory setting (psychological or otherwise). In a scientific laboratory you begin with a deliberate delimiting of extraneous variables in order to study and capture the desired variable. Although the goal is greater truth of the object, the method is to begin by decreasing the truth of the object. Everything is subtracted except the desired variable, which in turn—and just because of the deliberate narrowing of attention—can be studied all the more intensely.

In order to get more knowledge, we start with less. We shrink the world to a toy model; we study and expand our knowledge of only one variable. We then blow up the toy model back to real life size. We take the expanded variable and put it back into the true scale, real life world. Notice we are assuming that we are making no mistakes (no distortions) in our various manipulations and transformations of the real world (of course, we often do). Now, if all goes according to plan and we have correctly placed the expanded variable back into the true scale, real world, we really have increased our knowledge. Again, notice how many things have to go right for this to transpire, and how easy it is for a misfiring.

Perhaps, the psychoanalytic situation when it works, works analogously. That is, it begins with a radical delimiting of a whole, normal, dynamic, human relationship. It does this in order to dispel interfering variables so as to focus heightened abnormal attention on intrapsychic and interpersonal disturbances. It might well be, because of this initial delimiting, that whenever subsequent growth occurs (expansion and enrichment of intrapsychic, interpersonal, and developmental relating) it is at least partially caused by this. So far so good.

Yet here is where the double bind comes in: the patient does not *know* this, even if he knows it intellectually. What he basically experiences for a long time is instead the *delimiting* of the analytic situation. It is a delimiting that takes the special form of juxtaposing human relationship variables (professional technique and intimacy) that experientially do not belong together and therefore put him into a double bind that both puzzles and erodes his sense of interpersonal reality. As analysts, it may be more expedient to focus on the fruits, the payoff of our artificial, human laboratory experiment and to use it as a justification for the ongoing, powerful double bind that is one price tag, among others, for our patients' progress.

If the double bind arises from defiance of a cultural injunction against grossly conflicting levels of intimacy (technique and intimacy) we can ask where that cultural injunction comes from. Could there be an ethological injunction as well—an evolutionary, biological bias toward reciprocity in intimate relationships and *against* nonreciprocal intimacy, outside of familial settings?

This would be something like an evolutionary biological underpinning to the often heard warning to our children, "Do not take candy or gifts from strangers" (i.e., to not be easily intimate with strangers). If we think about it, the adaptive, biological survival value of infants and children responding naturally to an asymmetrical, but intimate bonding with their parents is obvious (Spitz 1965). It is also not difficult to see that if there should somehow be an ethological bias for resisting nonreciprocal, nonfamilial intimate, adult relationships (Spitz 1965, p. 150)—that is, for not lowering our defenses and readily conferring trust to a stranger, then this might also enhance species survival.

From the standpoint of the analytic situation, however, it makes no difference whatsoever whether the double bind is culturally or ethologically acquired. The main conflict is not one of paradoxical, mixed messages and conflicting levels of communication. It is one of paradoxical, conflicting levels of intimacy. The main inequity may not be one of power and control (as the double bind theorists have it), but one of nonreciprocal intimacy. This is not to deny the power gulf between analyst and patient (the rights, privileges, functions each enjoy) is substantial. It is to say *we seem to be able to tolerate a power inequity provided there is not also an intimacy inequity.*

This may be why we can accept doctors' and surgeons' vast power over our bodies and lives, comforted in the knowledge that the relationship (from the standpoint of intimacy) is impersonal on both sides. This may be why infants and children can accept, find nurturing, and naturally respond to an almost total power inequity between themselves and their parents, provided they sense a mutuality of love (reciprocal intimacy). By contrast, as analysts we know too well the lifelong, psychic scars that can accrue from a childhood perception of nonreciprocal, parental intimacy, i.e., parental power being used narcissistically or manipulatively, instead of lovingly.

Finally, we can return once again to the artist as perhaps the sole analogue in our culture wherein technique and intimacy (objectivity and subjectivity) can meet. The difference, of course, is that in the artist we are talking about a single, narcissistic process and a single person. It is one thing to have your subjectivity (intimacy) scrutinized by your objectivity (technique)—difficult though this may be in the case of the artist—when both subjectivity and objectivity are various aspects of a unitary self. It is quite another matter when your subjectivity and objectivity are divided up, not between yourself (as in the case of the artist), but between yourself and a stranger as in the case of the analytic situation. Here, personal objectivity is removed from the aegis of the self, and is externalized and placed into the hands of a powerful, professional stranger. This is a much more intimidating situation from the standpoint of the privacy and autonomy of the self, and one which can naturally give rise to the double bind.

THE FIRST THERAPEUTIC DOUBLE STANDARD

The founder of psychoanalysis may have been the first person to experience the untenable nature of the analytic double bind. In his revealing reminiscence of an analysis with Freud, Joseph Wortis (1954) reports when he asked Freud why he himself had never entered analysis, Freud suggested that, as founder, he may perhaps have been entitled to an exemption.

We can see that for what it was, a persuasive rationalization. Instead, perhaps what Freud was encountering, in addition to his own unanalyzed resistance, was a resistance to the pain of the analytic double bind and an understandable mystification at how to resolve it. It was relatively simple for Freud as a patriarchal, medical analyst to impart to his patients the injunction to free associate without censoring. Yet when it came time for himself to adopt his own analysand's rule (and thereby switch power and intimacy roles) he may have been at a loss as to how to do it. He was unable to relinquish the autonomy and self-esteem as founder to a disciple, perhaps feeling it was a contradiction and denial of his sense of self.

What he did not see, was that this contradiction existed *within* the psychoanalytic situation as well and did not simply pertain to the person of the founder. It pertained to every adult, intelligent, sensitive patient who is being asked to surrender a significant portion of his precious autonomy of self, now, in order to gain (later) a greater autonomy. It is irrelevant whether psychoanalysis pays off on this promise. Emotionally, it is experienced as a self-contradictory deprivation and a double bind. Freud, by asking for personal exemption as the founder, was really asking for *special pleading from a double bind he was unable to honor in practice, but only in theory.*

In one way, it can attest to the power of the double bind that it managed to discourage even Freud who could not find a way to deal with it. Looked at in this sense, self-analysis, whether by Freud (1900), or by his followers, may be an attempt to resolve the double bind of traditional psychoanalysis in the not-too-convincing, but emotionally reassuring way of having your cake and eating it, too. It may be a way of saying, Yes, I am being psychoanalyzed, but it is I who am doing the analysis; so it is I who has the control. As exempted founder, Freud could theoretically sweep away his need to enter psychoanalysis, making himself, perhaps, the only neurotic man on earth who did not have to go. He could as imperiously wave away every other patient's (basically similar) complaints about the loss of power, prestige, and autonomy as mere "resistance." Certainly without meaning to, Freud may have helped set the precedent for the *first therapeutic double standard.*

He may as well have set a precedent for psychoanalysis to underrate the pain, unending puzzlement, self-contradiction, the running counter to all cultural, social common sense—in short, the double bind of psychoanalysis—that has still not been fully resolved. Neo-Freudians and revisionists have at best only modified the double bind. At worst they have denied there is no easy short cut around it. We *have* to have professionalism, objectivity, the frame, neutrality, fee for service. We also have to have continuously candid self-disclosure and intimate psychic bonding on the part of the patient in order to have exploratory psychotherapy.

It may be other therapies have been motivated in part by an attempt to either resolve or escape outright from the double bind. From the psychoanalytic perspective, this can be seen as a *flight from the double bind*. It may have something to do with why so many patients pursue the panacea of psychotropic medication and much prefer it to the ordeal of analytic therapy. Besides the standard reasons—for example, gravity of the illness, eagerness or necessity for fast, symptomatic relief, search for a cure-all—may be a need for flight from the pain and conflicts of the double binds of analytic therapy.

The psychiatric patient may really be opting for a simple, doctor–patient model. In other words, don't work on my psyche, work on my biochemistry. You can have control of my neurotransmitters, but do not touch my sense of autonomy or sense of self. From the standpoint of analytic double binds it works fine. The price tag, of course, is large. There can be no hope of dynamic, exploratory psychotherapy and should the psychiatrist rule out medication and prescribe dynamic psychotherapy instead (as some do), the patient is right back in the double bind soup.

Perhaps part of the charm and current rage for Eriksonian (Jackson, p. 89) hypnotic or strategic, therapeutic techniques is that they promise to bypass the analytic double bind. The patient has only to passively submit, knowingly or unknowingly allowing his autonomy to be circumscribed as the master therapist (utilizing his metaphorical, neurolinguistic magic) speaks directly to his unconscious. The price tag is as high as in the doctor–patient model. In order to reap the benefits of highly directive, strategic therapy the patient must commence therapy by forsaking any real hope of consolidating his autonomy. If such patients enter therapy without the expectation of gaining a greater level of intimate relating, the double bind is to a great extent sidestepped. It is as though such patients and their therapists assume the black box idea of their illness and its treatment: it has almost nothing to do with them. By adopting as *impersonal* an idea of therapy as possible and, so to speak, putting themselves wholly in their therapists' hands, they may be also attempting to completely avoid double bind issues surrounding intimacy and control.

By contrast, existential psychotherapists may be trying to circumvent the double bind from an entirely different direction. By focusing so single-mindedly on meaning, they may be endeavoring to defend against the perceived *meaninglessness* of the analytic situation (i.e., the double bind that, to some extent, will always disturbingly run counter to common sense).

Transference and the Double Bind

We differ from double bind theorists (Jackson and Haley 1963) who see transference as a kind of externally, manipulatively induced form of childishness. On the other hand, it is useful to look at transference from the standpoint of the double bind, as not just the outcome of regressive illness or projective reaction to objects (internal, external). From the standpoint of the double bind, then, the analytic situation is not a tenable position. This means that once a patient is put into it, forces within will immediately conspire to get him out of it (in spite of any countering, positive transference or therapeutic alliance). This is because psychoanalysis, in just one of its revolutionary side effects, came up with the idea of joining—in a way never before done—two very strange bedfellows: technique and intimacy. Since they never have gotten along well together, it was inevitable there would be immediate affects and effects, forcing a (necessary) emotional clash and dialogue.

To understand the connection between the double bind and

transference, it is revealing to look at just what transference accomplishes. Again, just from the standpoint of the double bind, transference does a lot. Transference takes a professional relationship and transforms it into an intensely intimate relationship. Transference takes two strangers who have only just met and transforms them into lifelong, blood relatives. It takes two incompatible levels of intimacy and makes them both complementary and reciprocal (even if negatively so). It can thereby still the anxiety that one is opening up one's intimacy before a professional stranger who may turn out to be cold-blooded; to be vengeful; to be critical; to be indifferent; to be interested in using the patient only for monetary gain. It does this, it rescues the patient by pulling out from the terrifying void of professional estrangement something even more magically familiar than a friend—a parent or sibling.

Seen in this light, transference accomplishes a lot. Because so much attention has been paid to its infantile roots, its skillfulness has probably not been given sufficient credit. Yet, looked at strictly and only from the vantage point of the double bind, we can sum it up by saying: *Transference (apart from everything else attributed to it) is restitution and denial. It is a magical attempt to resolve the double bind of nonreciprocal intimacy by substituting for the actual analytic relationship an early parent/sibling–child imago which is far more reassuringly representative of reciprocal intimacy (and this is so even if the transference is negative).*

To summarize: the concept of the double bind has mainly flourished in the family system therapies. By contrast, it has been overlooked by psychoanalytic therapists. It is suggested that the double bind, while not often seen as important as the intrapsychic or interpersonal factors, is certainly real. A concept of the analytic double bind has been presented. The analytic double bind is not one of paradoxical, mixed messages and conflicting levels of communication. Instead, it arises from a conflict of incompatible levels of intimacy—specifically, the conflict between technique and intimacy. Finally, an attempt has been made to delineate this central double bind both from the viewpoint of the analyst and from the viewpoint of the patient.

Conclusion

Making It

Although the odds are long, and stacked against them, some young artists do make it.

Steve, the pianist who seemed able to magically metamorphose while performing, was one who did. About a year after he stopped therapy, he returned to New York and paid me an unexpected visit. He had just concluded a highly successful concert tour throughout Europe. There had been rave reviews. He was negotiating with a producer from a record company who was eager to sign him up. He had just given a private performance for a famous conductor who had immediately asked him to play a concerto, as part of an upcoming, major AIDS benefit.

Leaning boyishly forward from the edge of the couch, trying to look composed and mature, although I could tell his mind was racing, Steve wanted to tell me all this and more. He had been winning and expecting to win piano competitions ever since he was eight years old, but he had never cashed in before. Not this big. As I listened, I couldn't help remembering his amazing debut as a solo pianist in New York City. He had been poor then and relatively unknown, and now he was rapidly getting famous and on his way to becoming rich. But what struck me was, he didn't seem (psychologically) that different.

And in the few instances, where poor struggling artists managed to become successful and recognized, this was borne out. Success, when it finally came, seemed to leave a very different impact upon the artist, than it did upon the nonartist. In the case of the artist, success, rather than the consolidation and attainment of a higher rung in a sanctioned ladder of achievement, more often resembled a manic interlude, a burst of energy, or an inspiration. But an inspiration on the part of the public who had mysteriously been moved to embrace someone it had previously been content to ignore. Recognition conferred upon artists fundamentally differs from recognition given to nonartists inasmuch as it is not based on accepted progress in completion of a traditional role but is connected to the degree of narcissistic gratification perceived by the audience. Artists, therefore, are sooner or later forced to accept they are only as good as their last hit, and their reputation no less transient than their popularity.

Since artists measure so much of their self-esteem by the yardstick of their creative actualization, and since creativity is such an inherently unstable state of dynamic change and flux, their identities are correspondingly often unfinished, problematical, and needy of constant reassurance and proving. Although ego-functions are essential to the implementation of creative goals (and their impairment is often the main reason they enter therapy), artists know without a fertile, vital, and more than fleeting contribution from their unconscious there is little hope of success.

Compared with a physician or lawyer, no licensing procedure, ritualistic diploma or certification, exists for an artist. By contrast, a lawyer who passes a bar exam and a physician who graduates from medical school are a lawyer and a physician for life. No such rite of passage—regardless of the degree of success achieved—exists for the artist, whose recognition tends to be dependent upon the narcissistic gratification he delivers. They are therefore judged on a need-gratifying, immediacy basis—that is to say, strictly by their present performance. Because of this, unless they are actively engaged in the process of gratifying their real or imaginary audience, it is hard for artists to feel they are artists, regardless of past successes. And since success is rarely found in the portfolio of young artists, they are that much more fearful of being unable to follow-up in a solid way any serendipitous creative triumphs.

The Young Artist as Prototype

The young artist who makes it (as was the case with Steve and others) is susceptible to a kind of artistic paranoia, manifested by feelings of depression which often alternate with the manic interlude of first success. It is caused, in part, by a dread that even if he has correctly read the mind and mood of his audience (who are notoriously fickle), there is always a very good chance the tide can change. Accordingly, artists, once the roar of success dies down, often nervously return to their drawing boards to make sure they have their aesthetic mechanics down pat. No matter how successful he can become, the young struggling artist who preceded him is never very far away and for that reason—to my mind—is the real prototype of the more mature artist whom the public eventually gets to know.

The splits, double binds, paradoxes, inhibitions, mistrust, conflicts over intimacy, the narcissism and paranoia that have been portrayed are sometimes the price and barriers to what they are trying to do. It is not meant to diminish the value of who they are or what they are attempting. The value of that endeavor is not to be found in the customary indices of prestige and success, nor by a cool measurement of the weight of their subsequent accomplishments.

They are better understood by looking at the nature of their struggle and the depth of their vision with which they start out. What do young artists want? Among other things, to express as much of what is most human about themselves in as potent, enduring, and beautiful a symbolism as they can create.

At a time of vanishing personal frontiers, when the most acclaimed loners tend to be celebrities, sports heroes, or romantic gangsters, the young struggling artist remains often misunderstood, admirable, not infrequently a splendid underdog, and on occasion even—to use an old-fashioned word—noble.

Glossary

While the book is intended for both the professional and lay reader, the glossary is aimed at the nonspecialist. The terms that are included are those which are not fully explained in the text, and, whenever I depart from a standard definition, I try to provide my reasons for doing so.

abreaction A notion which derives from Freud's early work on the causation and genesis of hysterical symptoms. It refers to the emotional discharge whereby a person frees himself from the affect (emotion) attached to the memory of a traumatic event so as to prevent the affect from becoming capable of producing pathology. Freud's idea was that unless such painful affects were discharged, whether through psychotherapy or spontaneous associative draining off, they would accumulate in the unconscious and eventually manifest themselves in the form of a hysterical symptom.

as-if personality Associated with the psychoanalyst Helene Deutsch. It describes a type of passive, schizoid person who severs emotional bonds when it comes to relating to other people, who searches the environment for cues as how to appropriately behave and then does his best to "stage" the desirable performance. Although considered somewhat rare, the as-if personality is an example of a psychological designation that has filtered into the contemporary consciousness, in no small part, because it has been so memorably named.

catharsis A Greek word meaning purification or purging and used by Aristotle to explain the effect tragedy produces on the spectator. When used in psychotherapy, it is a method in which the therapeutic effect sought is purgative: that is, there is an appropriate discharge of emotions which have become fixated on traumatic past experiences.

denial An unconscious defense mechanism whereby emotions or ideas that are gauged to be too tension-producing or threatening to be safely incorporated or integrated, are dealt with by dismissal, which can be seen as an attempt to expel or banish the unwelcome intruder from the conscious realm of approved beliefs. Since denial, according to psychoanalytic theory, operates unconsciously, it is not to be confused with disagreement, discrimination, or debate, which can be predominantly a conscious, cognitive phenomenon. Compared with repression, which can entail the blotting out of an entire experience, denial is extremely economical so far as defense mechanisms go. It can admit into consciousness every detail, thought, and feeling of a given experience—providing it somehow (unconsciously) finds a way to dispute the final validity or particular inference that someone is drawing. Thus, denial kind of pulls the rug out from reality. It is perhaps best and most poignantly seen in the person who has just been apprised that he is the victim of a terminal illness, who will often—after accepting every piece of medical evidence and data his doctor can bring to bear—manages to conclude, "Yes, but I am *not* going to die."

To the therapist who must be professionally alert to the appearance and machinations of all kinds of defensive operations, denial is an especially vivid and widespread defense mechanism.

depersonalization The state of feeling robbed of one's personal attributes (objectified, turned into an object) or the activity of turning another person into such an object. It can arise in many ways, but one of the most common is as the end result of a defensive operation by which one either withdraws or aggressively attacks certain qualities of human intimacy which are perceived as threatening.

derealization The complement of depersonalization; however, applied to the perception of reality. Feelings of derealization are often expressed as, "This can't be real," "This can't be happening." The persistence of such feelings can be one indication of a schizoid personality.

double bind This is associated with the work of Gregory Bateson, who sought to discover the genesis of schizophrenia within the interpersonal network of family dynamics. A double bind was considered to be comprised of three elements: (1) an incompatibility of conflicting levels of communication (mixed messages); (2) a legitimate threat attached to each of the mixed messages—thus, a "damned if you do and damned if you don't" scenario is achieved; and (3) a prohibition (to the person pinned in the double bind) to either leave the specific field of interpersonal conflict, or to comment on it. The cumulative effect of such family-inspired double binds, according to Bateson, was schizophrenia. Although psychoanalytic theory has largely passed over double binds, I believe it deserves more attention than it has received. However, in contrast to the traditional double bind theorists, I conceive the primary double bind—instead of a conflict between incongruent levels of communication—to arise as an irreconcilable clash between incompatible levels of relating, specifically, between technique and intimacy. And I consider the artistic temperament, with its inevitable mismatch of spontaneous creativity coupled with an intense need to symbolically orchestrate such outpourings, to be a fertile breeding ground for numerous double binds.

empathy A capacity to experience the feelings and subjective experience of another person ("to put oneself in someone else's shoes"). It is not to be confused with sympathy. In the book, I try to characterize the importance of empathy by comparing it with its opposite: the-not-having-a-clue as to what the other person is thinking and feeling which (in the extreme case of the paranoid) can result in distortions of inhuman and monstrous persecutions.

false self Often associated with the writings of D. W. Winnicott. It is meant to describe a fragmentation in the ego of certain compliant patients who erect a false, as-if persona which they use as a defensive shield to protect the presumed fragile true self from fantasized dangers. I apply Winnicott's important classification, not to patients, but to the analyst himself, the analytic technique, and the analytic situation.

grandiose self Primarily associated with the work of Heinz Kohut, the term is meant to evoke an early stage in the development of the psyche in which there is an intense, primitive, unrealistic, exhibitionistic, and inflated self-involvement. Unless the grandiose self is subsequently integrated into a more adaptive self-esteem (what Kohut would consider healthy narcissism), it could become a source of future pathology.

intellectualization A defense mechanism that seeks to force a posture of disciplined understanding upon unconscious thoughts and feelings that are felt to be disturbingly out of control. By tenaciously insisting that one's behavior is only the product of thorough cognitive processing, an attempt is made to secure a sense of power and predictability that is considered necessary.

narcissism In Freud's seminal work of 1914, he conceived of an original state in which the infant, who has not yet learned to differentiate, conceptualize, or relate to an object, invests his primitive pleasure ego in aspects of himself. Freud called this stage a primary narcissism (self-love) and he considered it a normal stepping stone to a higher, developmental love, object love (or love of another person). Sometimes, however, there is a fixation or only partial resolution to the early stage of primary narcissism and what results is the character disorder called a narcissistic personality—someone who is self-involved, self-invested, and self-loving to an abnormal degree. To the modern, who often insatiably pursues self-sustaining and self-validating aims, the term can ring strangely true, and, in certain respects, the idea of narcissism has become one of the paradigmatic illnesses of our time.

narcissistic injury Anything that threatens or is taken to diminish the exaggerated standards of self-regard of the narcissist. Typically, narcissists are hypersensitive to anything that does not embellish their sense of themselves, that does not make them feel good, powerful, or loved.

narcissistic personality Compulsive sexual seducers (Don Juans); compulsively aggressive, intrusive people (high-pressure salesmen); exhibitionistic types (actors) are often lumped together as specific examples of a general narcissistic personality. In the book, instead of treating the unquestionable narcissism of artists as derivative of an underlying personality disturbance, I regard their extraordinary creativity as a kind of narcissistic persona in itself, capable of producing and explaining a good deal of the observed dynamics of the artistic temperament.

obsessional doubt or uncertainty A displaced and symptomatic expression of an underlying conflict, often involving an ambivalence (love/hate) of feeling toward another person. According to psychoanalytic theory, the central ambivalence of feeling is repressed and displaced onto a much less threatening ambivalence; e.g., in the case of the obsessional doubter, a compulsion to find the answer to essentially unanswerable questions (the meaning of life, speculations about the nature of death, etc.).

paranoia Classified as a psychosis. In classical psychoanalytic theory, it was considered the outcome of a complicated process of denial, transformation, and projection of repressed homosexual impulses onto another person. In the book, I treat paranoia from a phenomenological standpoint (which is not to deny the important dynamics of its etiology), and I regard it as a defense mainly against *intimacy* (which may or may not include homosexual intimacy).

paranoid style Primarily associated with David Shapiro and his classic *Neurotic Styles* (1965). The paranoid style refers to the characterological way in which a typical paranoid relates to his inner and outer world. In the sense that it does not traditionally focus on isolated symptoms as a defense against an underlying, presumed nuclear conflict, it is a holistic approach.

projection A major defensive operation of the mind which seeks to avoid pain by converting threatening or overwhelming inner stimuli to outer ones. It thereby creates distance and safety between the ego and what the ego fears. The person who projects—by transforming ambiguous, disturbing inner affects or ideas to a specific point in external reality—now has the option of either successfully fleeing or aggressively attacking the perceived, visible threat. There is a second sense in which projection is used: the tendency of the mind to organize reality, especially undifferentiated reality, according to the structure of the individual personality. Thus, each person has a unique style of perceiving and organizing reality which, when faced with amorphous cues such as ink blots on a Rorschach test, projects itself onto the material at hand. Such is the rationale underlying projective testing.

projective identification In projection, what is projected is usually experienced as alien or at least differentiated from the ego of the person who projects (otherwise, what is the point of projecting?). In projective identification, however, after an initial expulsion of undesirable content from the unconscious of the person, there is a subsequent identification with what has previously been expelled. It is as though—now that the safety factor of distance has been added—it is no longer threatening to identify with the psychical contents, so long as they are perceived to be comfortably residing in another person's psyche. In this sense, projective identification may be considered a midpoint or compromise between identification and projection.

rationalization A defense mechanism whereby the ego—in an attempt to explain its behavior to itself—selects from a series of coexisting motives the one that seems most sensible and rational. The adaptive value of this should be obvious: the ego is spared from internal recriminations, anxiety, or guilt from perceived faulty behavior, while simultaneously warding off possible external criticism.

repression A universal defensive operation of the mind which seeks to bar from consciousness psychical stimuli that are considered too painful to bear. Repression works in a variety of ways—dissociation of affect and thought, displacement, condensation, disguise, denial, symptom formation—but the aim is the same: to protect the ego from harm. Freud distinguished between normal repression, repression that results in the formation of neurotic symptoms, the return of the repressed, rerepression, and failure of repression resulting, for example, in the outbreak of frankly psychotic behavior.

schizoid personality Someone who is extremely passive, out of touch, disconnected, and dissociated from his feelings, and who exhibits various splits between his thoughts, feelings, and behavior.

selfobject Derived from the work of Heinz Kohut. It describes an early stage in the development of normal narcissism in which an external object (person) is used as a bulwark to a fragile sense of self-love. A selfobject is therefore an external person who is treated as though he were a literal extension of the subject's sense of self. Kohut articulates this with the sentences "You are perfect. But I am part of you." The advantage of treating another person as a part of one's self is that it confers a comforting (although false) sense of control and power over that person, while effectively denying his autonomy. There are few things more unpleasant than to be dealt with as only an appendage of someone else's psyche. Kohut regarded the use of selfobjects as a stage to be surmounted in the establishment of healthy narcissism or appropriate self-esteem. I use the term *objective selfobject* to designate the unique linkage that exists between the artist and an external confirming audience—a symbiotic bond which, by the nature of the artistic process, is never really surmounted or relinquished.

splitting of the ego Late in his life, Freud conceived of splitting as a radical defensive maneuver of the ego. Splitting is a way of almost simultaneously relating in two incompatible ways. The advantage is that the person, so to speak, can have his cake and eat it, too. The disadvantage is that in splitting, the ego must sacrifice the synthesizing function that is its hallmark.

symbiosis In biology, this occurs when two different species (e.g., a host and a parasite) have their life cycles unalterably linked. In psychoanalysis, it refers to an interdependence of two separate people who biologically are capable of living apart, but—because of a pathological psychological dependency—are unable to do so.

true self The counterpart of the false self, and also derived from D. W. Winnicott. The true self is meant to evoke the creative, spontaneous, alive core of the person's essence that, unfortunately, is often perceived as being too precious and brittle to be put on display, and is therefore camouflaged. As with the false self, I apply this concept, not to patients, but to the analyst himself, the analytic technique, and the analytic situation.

References

Alper, G. 1990. The double bind in psychoanalysis. *The Journal of Contemporary Psychotherapy,* **20**(4): 273–282.

Barrett, W. 1979. *The illusion of technique.* Garden City, NY: Anchor Press/Doubleday.

———. 1982. *The truant's adventures among the intellectuals.* New York: Anchor Press/Doubleday.

Bateson, G.; Jackson, D. D.; Haley, J.; and Weakland J. H. 1956. Toward a theory of schizophrenia. In *Communication, family and marriage,* Vol. 1, Human Communication Series, edited by Don D. Jackson. Palo Alto, CA: Science and Behavior Books.

Bion, W. R. 1970. *Attention and interpretation.* London: Tavistock Publications.

———. 1977. *Two papers: The grid and caesura.* Rio de Janeiro: Imago Editora.

———. 1974. *Experiences in groups.* New York: Basic Books.

———. 1975. *Attention and interpretation.* London: Tavistock.

Deutsch, H. 1942. Some forms of emotional disturbance and their relationship to schizophrenia. In *Neuroses and character types.* New York: International Universities Press.

———. 1990. *Brazilian lectures*. London: H. Karnac (Books).
Edelson, M. 1984. *Hypothesis and evidence in psychoanalysis*. Chicago and London: The University of Chicago Press.
Erikson, E. H. 1959. *Identity and the life cycle*. Psychological Issues, No. 1. New York: International Universities Press.
Feynman, R. P. 1985. *QED: The strange theory of light and matter*. Princeton, NJ: Princeton University Press.
Freud, S. 1895. *Project for a scientific psychology*. Standard Edition, 1:281–397. London: Hogarth Press, 1966.
———. 1895. *Studies on hysteria*. Standard Edition, 22, London: Hogarth Press, 1957.
———. 1900. *The interpretation of dreams*.Standard Edition, 4 & 5. London: Hogarth Press, 1953.
———. 1908. *The relation of the poet to day-dreaming*. In *Collected papers*, 4:173–183. London: Hogarth Press, 1946.
———. 1909. *Notes upon a case of obsessional neurosis*. Standard Edition, 10:155. London: Hogarth Press, 1957.
———. 1910. *Leonardo da Vinci and a memory of his childhood*. Standard Edition, 9. London: Hogarth Press, 1957.
———. 1911a. *Formulations on the two principles of mental functioning*. Standard Edition, 12:218–226. London: Hogarth Press, 1958.
———. 1911b. *Psycho-analytic notes on an autobiographical account of a case of paranoia*. Standard Edition, 3. London: Hogarth Press, 1958.
———. 1914. *On narcissism: An introduction*. Standard Edition, 14:73–102. London: Hogarth Press, 1957.
———. 1915. *Repression*. Standard Edition, 14:146–158. London: Hogarth Press, 1957.
———. 1922. *Group psychology and the analysis of the ego*. Standard Edition, 18:65–143. London: Hogarth Press, 1961.
———. 1923. *The ego and the id*. Standard Edition, 19:3. London: Hogarth Press, 1961.
———. 1926. *The problem of anxiety*. Standard Edition, 20:77. London: Hogarth Press, 1959.
———. 1928. *The future of an illusion*. Standard Edition, 21. London: Hogarth Press, 1974.
———. 1938. *Splitting of the ego in the process of defense*. Standard Edition, 23:271–279. London: Hogarth Press, 1964.
Gleick, J. 1987. *Chaos*. New York: Viking Penguin.
Greenberg, J. 1964. *I never promised you a rose garden*. New York: Holt, Rinehart and Winston.

References

Haley, J. 1958. An interactional explanation of hypnosis. In *Therapy, communication, and change,* edited by Don D. Jackson. Vol. 1, Human Communication Series. Palo Alto, CA: Science and Behavior Books, 1968.

Heidegger, M. 1968. *What is called thinking?* New York: Harper & Row.

Herbert, N. 1987. *Quantum reality beyond the new physics.* New York: Anchor Press/Doubleday.

Jackson, D. D., and Haley, J. 1963. Transference revisited. In *Therapy, communication, and change,* edited by Don D. Jackson. pp. 115–129. Vol. 1, Human Communication Series. Palo Alto, CA: Science and Behavior Books, 1968.

Janik, A., and Toulmin, S. 1973. *Wittgenstein's Vienna.* New York: Simon and Schuster.

Kernberg, O. 1975. Borderline personality organization; The treatment of the narcissistic personality; Clinical problems of the narcissistic personality; and Normal and pathological narcissism. In *Borderline conditions and pathological narcissism.* New York: Jason Aronson.

———. 1986. Technical strategies in the treatment of narcissistic personalities. In *Severe personality disorders psychotherapeutic strategies.* New Haven and London: Yale University Press.

———. 1987. Projection and projective identification: Developmental and clinical aspects. In *Projection, identification, projective identification.* Madison, CT: International Universities Press.

Khan, M. M. R. 1974. Clinical aspects of the schizoid personality: Affects and technique. In *The privacy of the self.* London: The Hogarth Press.

———. 1979. *Alienation in perversions.* New York: International Universities Press.

———. 1981. *The privacy of the self.* London: Hogarth Press.

Klein, M. 1946. Notes on some schizoid mechanisms. In *Developments in psychoanalysis,* edited by J. Riviére. London: Hogarth Press.

Kohut, H. 1971. *The analysis of the self.* New York: International Universities Press.

———. 1977. *The restoration of the self.* New York: International Universities Press.

Kris, E. 1950. On preconscious mental processes. *Psychoanalytic Quarterly* **19**: 540–560.

Krystal, H. 1973. Self representation and the capacity for self care. In *The annual of psychoanalysis,* Vol. 6. New York: International Universities Press, pp. 209–247, GA.

Kübler-Ross, E. 1969. *On death and dying.* New York: Collier Books/Macmillan.
Laing, R. D. 1961. *Self and others.* London: Tavistock Publications.
———. 1970a. *The divided self.* Baltimore, MD: Penguin Books.
———. 1970b. *Knots.* New York: Pantheon Books.
———. 1982. *The voice of experience.* New York: Pantheon Books.
———; Phillipson, H.; and Lee, A. R. 1966. *Interpersonal perception: A theory and a method of research.* New York: Harper & Row.
Langs, R. 1976. *The therapeutic interaction,* Vols. 1 & 2. New York: Jason Aronson.
Lindner, R. 1954. The jet-propelled couch. In *The fifty-minute hour: A collection of true psychoanalytic tales.* New York: Delta.
Malcolm, N. 1958. *Ludwig Wittgenstein a memoir with a biographical sketch by Georg Henrik Von Wright.* New York: Oxford University Press.
Meissner, W. W. 1978. *The paranoid process.* New York: Jason Aronson.
———. 1987. Projection and projective identification. In *Projection, identification, projective identification.* Madison, CT: International Universities Press.
Miller, A. 1981. *The drama of the gifted child.* New York: Basic Books.
Pears, D. 1969. *Ludwig Wittgenstein.* New York: Viking Press.
Popper, K. R., and Eccles, J. C. 1977. *The self and its brain.* London: Routledge & Kegan Paul.
Pribram, K. H., and Gill, M. M. 1976. *Freud's "project" reassessed.* New York: Basic Books.
Racker, H. 1968. *Transference and counter-transference.* New York: International Universities Press.
Rapaport, D. 1976. *The collected papers of David Rapaport.* New York: Basic Books.
Ricoeur, P. 1970. *Freud and philosophy: An essay on interpretation.* New Haven, CT: Yale University Press.
Roth, P. 1970. *My life as a man.* New York: Penguin Books.
Sandler, J. 1987a. *Projection, identification, projective identification.* Madison, CT: International Universities Press.
———. 1987b. The concept of projective identification. In *Projection, identification, projective identification.* Madison, CT: International Universities Press.
Sandler, J., and Rosenblatt, B. 1962. The concept of the representational world. *The Psychoanalytic Study of the Child,* **17**:128–145. New York: International Universities Press.

References

Sartre, J. 1956. *Being and nothingness.* New York: Simon and Schuster.
Schafer, R. 1976. *A new language for psychoanalysis.* New Haven, CT: Yale University Press.
———. 1979. *The analytic attitude.* New York: Basic Books.
Schur, M. 1972. *Freud: Living and dying.* New York: International Universities Press.
Searles, H. 1960. *The nonhuman environment.* New York: International Universities Press.
———. 1979. *Countertransference and related subjects.* New York: International Universities Press.
Shapiro, D. 1965. *Neurotic styles.* New York: Basic Books.
Spitz, R. A. 1965. *The first year of life.* New York: International Universities Press.
Stolorow, R. D.; Brandchaft, B.; and Atwood, G. 1987. *Psychoanalytic treatment: An intersubjective approach.* Hillsdale, NJ: The Analytic Press.
Sullivan,H. S. 1973. *Clinical studies in psychiatry.* New York: W. W. Norton.
Vonnegut, K. 1965. *God bless you, Mr. Rosewater.* New York: Dell.
———. 1982. *Slaughterhouse five.* New York: Dell.
Whitehead, A. N., and Russell, B. 1962. *Principia mathematica.* Cambridge, U.K.: Cambridge University Press.
Winnicott, D. W. 1953. Transitional objects and transitional phenomena. *International Journal of Psychoanalysis,* Vol. 34.
———. 1958. Clinical varieties of transference. In *Collected papers: Through paediatrics to psychoanalysis.* London: Tavistock.
———. 1960. Ego distortion in terms of true and false self. In *The maturational processes and the facilitating environment.* New York: International Universities Press.
Wittgenstein, L. 1922. *Tractatus logico-philosophicus.* London: Routledge & Kegan Paul.
———. 1953. *Philosophical investigations.* New York: Macmillan.
———. 1956. *Remarks on the foundations of mathematics.* Oxford, U.K.: Basil Blackwell.
———. 1958. *The blue and brown books.* New York: Harper & Row.
———. 1969. *On certainty.* New York: Harper & Row.
———. 1972. *Lectures and conversations on aesthetics, psychology and religious belief,* ed. C. Barrett. Berkeley and Los Angeles: University of California Press.

———. 1977. *Remarks on colour*. Berkeley and Los Angeles: University of California Press.

Wortis, J. 1954. *Fragments of an analysis with Freud*. New York: Simon and Schuster.

Index

Abreaction, 84, 85
 definition, 221
 linguistic, 173
Actors
 case example, 31–43
 creativity of, 22
 employment as waiters, 22–24
 therapeutic double bind of, 21–22
Aggression, in therapist–patient relationship, 191–193
Alcoholics Anonymous (A.A.), 61
Alienation, 146
Analyst. *See* Therapist
Analytic situation. *See also* Therapist–patient relationship
 delimitation of, 207–208
 interpersonal falseness of, 185–

Analytical situation (*cont.*)
 191, 197
 intimacy in, 208–209
 laboratory setting analogy, 206–209
Anxiety, therapy-related, 193
Aristotle, 222
Artists
 compliance of, 154, 156
 cultural attitudes toward, 146–148, 149
 employment of, 22–26, 148
 false self, 26
 inner self, 154–156
As-if personality, 153, 154–155, 221–222
Atomism, logical, 164, 168
Audience–artist relationship, 12–15

Audience–artist relationship (*cont.*)
  as artist's primary relationship, 39–40
  audience as selfobject, 13, 15, 40
  detachment in, 149
  intimacy in, 17–19, 149
  narcissism in, 14–15, 18–19
  narcissistic injury in, 14, 15
  of performing artists, 14–15, 20
  receptivity in, 14
  sadomasochism of, 19–20
  self-esteem and, 12–13
  symbiotic nature of, 19–20
Autonomy, of patient, 211–212

Bateson, Gregory, 223
Beethoven, Ludwig Van, 40
Blocking, creative, 7, 148
Blue and Brown Books, The (Wittgenstein), 164
Bohr, Niels, 174
Buyer–seller relationship, narcissistic injury in, 24–26

Catharsis, 84, 85, 222
Charisma, 8
Code of conduct, of therapist, 191–194
Compliance, of the artist, 154, 156
Countertransference, 10–12
  with actors, 22
  with paranoid patients, 97
  with terminally ill patients, 109
  therapist's identity in, 205
  therapist's truthfulness in, 205
Creative blocking, 7, 148
Creativity
  of actors, 22

Creativity (*cont.*)
  hyperdevelopment of, 149–150
  narcissism and, 6, 18
  the unconscious and, 150–151
Cultural attitudes, toward artists, 146–148, 149

Death and dying
  defense mechanisms, 122–135
    adaptive defenses, 125, 126
    double bind and, 132–133
    ego splitting, 129–130
    intellectualization, 126–127
    paranoid defenses, 129
    projection, 127–129
    rationalization, 130–131
    repression, 131
    schizoid defenses, 130
  ego and, 132
  Freud's theory of, 133
  religious belief and, 133
Deemotionalization, of object relations, 153
Defense mechanisms
  against death, 122–135
    adaptive defenses, 125, 126
    double bind and, 132–133
    ego splitting, 129–130
    intellectualization, 126–127
    paranoid defenses, 129
    projection, 127–129
    rationalization, 130–131
    repression, 131
    schizoid defenses, 130
  narcissism as, 17, 18–19, 26
  of schizoid personality, 153
Delusional patient, 47–49
Denial
  of death, 222
  suicide as, 134

Index

Denial of death (*cont.*)
  by terminally ill patient, 113, 117, 118, 122–124, 127, 133
  definition, 222–223
  of narcissistic injury, 25–26
Depersonalization, 152–153, 155–156, 223
Depression
  creative blocking and, 7
  following creative effort, 6
  narcissistic, 16, 39
  of terminally ill patient, 101–103, 108, 111, 113
Derealization, 155, 223
Detachment, 146
Detective stories, paranoia of, 94
Deutsch, Helene, 221–222
Double bind
  of the artist, 36
  of audience–artist relationship, 15
  of death and dying, 132–133
  elements of, 223
  of family dynamics, 201, 202, 223
  therapeutic, 17–28, 223–224
    analytic situation and, 186
    artists' creativity and, 21–22
    financial factors in, 205–206
    Freud and, 209–211
    intimacy and, 17, 27–28, 92, 93–94, 203, 208–209, 213
    origins of, 202–203, 206–209
    paradox of, 28, 188
    of paranoid patients, 92–94
    psychotropic medication and, 211
    self-analysis and, 210
    therapeutic double standard and, 209–212

Double bind, therapeutic (*cont.*)
    therapeutic interpretation and, 152
    therapist's dilemma of, 204–206
    transference and, 212–213
Double standard, therapeutic, 209–212
Doubt, obsessional, 225–226
Douglas, Kirk, 23
Drug abuse
  creative effort and, 6–7
  by paranoid patients, 60–64
  trauma and, 64, 66–68
Dyson, Freeman, 167

Ego, death and, 132
Ego-ideal, 13, 21
Ego splitting, 9–10, 129–130, 228
Einstein, Albert, 174
Empathy
  definition, 224
  of imagination, 195
  of paranoid patients, 89–91
  of terminally ill patients, 124
Employment, of artists, 22–26, 148
Eriksonian therapy, 211–212
Existential psychotherapy, 212
Eye contact, with patient, 54–57

Falsifiability, of scientific hypotheses, 170
Family dynamics
  of double bind, 201, 202, 223
  libidinal, 20–21
Family system therapy, 201, 202
Fantasy
  paranoid, 49–52

Fantasy, paranoid (*cont.*)
  Freud's theory of, 85
  therapist's involvement in, 86–89
  of suicide, 79–81
Feynman, Richard, 28
Freud, Sigmund, 161
  death theory of, 133
  double bind and, 209–211
  group leader theory of, 13, 20–21
  Leonardo da Vinci study of, 160
  metapsychology of, 175
  narcissism theory of, 224–225
  paranoid fantasy theory of, 85
  prose style of, 171–173
  Wittgenstein and, 171–173

Genius, paranoid style and, 168–169
Gestalt therapy, 189–190
Godfather, The (film), 96–97
Grandiosity, 78–79, 146
Grateful Dead, 65–67
Gratification, narcissistic, 218–219
Group leader, 13, 20–21

Heisenberg, Werner, 174
Herbert, N., 174
Hypnotic therapy, 211–212
Hysteria, 84–85

Id, 130
Identity development, 9–10
Imagination, empathic, 195
I Never Promised You a Rose Garden (Green), 185
Inner self, of the artist, 154–156
Inspiration, artistic, 26–27, 148

Inspiration, artistic (*cont.*)
  therapeutic interpretation analogy, 151–152
Intellectualization, 126–127, 224
Interpersonal relationships, of artists, 39–40
  theatricality of, 40, 154–156
Intimacy
  of the artist, 209
  of audience–artist relationship, 17–19, 149
  of paranoid patients, 89–98
  in parent–child relationship, 208–209
  in therapeutic double bind, 17, 27–28, 92, 93–94, 203, 208–209, 213
  transference and, 213

Kindness, of therapist, 195–196
Kohut, Heinz, 40, 227, 228
Kraus, Karl, 161

Laing, R.D., 90, 189
Lancaster, Burt, 23
Language use
  psychoanalysts' use of, 169–173, 174–176
  trauma of, 165–166
  Wittgenstein's theory of, 163, 164, 165–166, 168–176
Life-style, artistic, 36, 42
Lindner, Robert, 48–49
Logical atomism, 164, 168
Logical positivism, 163, 164, 175
LSD, 66–68

Mean Streets (film), 63
Meissner, W.W., 88–89

Index

Metapsychology, psychoanalytic, 174–175
Moore, G.E., 162
Musicians, case examples, 3–5, 8
    paranoid, 47–48, 49–84, 86–90, 91–93, 96, 97–98
My Life as a Man (Roth), 56

Narcissism, 36
    in audience–artist relationship, 14–15, 18–19
    creativity and, 6, 18
    as defense mechanism, 17, 18–19, 26
    definition, 224–225
    depression and, 16, 39
    employment and, 22–26
    healthy, 40
    primary, 224–225
    self-esteem and, 40
Narcissistic defeat, 16
Narcissistic gratification, 218–219
Narcissistic injury
    in audience–artist relationship, 14, 15
    in buyer–seller relationship, 24–26
    definition, 225
    denial of, 25–26
    to paranoid patient, 82–83
Narcissistic personality, 225
Narcotics Anonymous, 60–61
Neorealism, 174
Neurotic Styles (Shapiro), 226
Nightmares, 23

Object choice, narcissistic, 27, 39
Object love, 225
Object relations, 155
    deemotionalization of, 153

On Certainty (Wittgenstein), 169

Painter, case example, 139–146, 150
Paranoia
    definition, 226
    following narcissistic depression, 39
    personality characteristics of, 166
    of popular culture, 94, 96–97
    of successful artists, 219
    transitional, 87
Paranoid patient, 47–98
    case example, 47–48, 49–84, 86–90, 91–93, 96, 97–98
    countertransference with, 97
    double bind of, 92–94
    drug abuse by, 60–64
    empathy of, 89–91
    eye contact with, 54–57
    grandiose thinking of, 78–79
    homosexual impulses of, 93–94
    hostility of, 91–92
    intimacy with, 89–98
    LSD use by, 66–68
    mistrust by, 96–97
    narcissistic injury to, 82–83
    paranoid episodes of, 70–75, 81–82, 87, 97
    paranoid thinking of, 84–86, 94, 95
    projection by, 90–91, 93
    projective testing of, 95
    psychiatric consultation for, 71, 76, 79, 97
    psychoanalytic historical method for, 77–78
    psychosis of, 87
    role reversal with, 87–88

Paranoid patient (*cont.*)
  suicidal fantasies of, 79–81
  termination of therapy by, 97–98
  therapeutic crisis of, 79
  therapist's ambivalence toward, 49–50
  therapist's paranoid alliance with, 86–89, 91
  transference with, 86, 97
  trust in therapist of, 75–76, 86
Paranoid process, 88–89, 161
Paranoid style, 226
Parent–child relationship
  as double bind situation, 202, 203–204
  intimacy in, 208–209
Peale, Norman Vincent, 8
Performing artists. *See also* Actors; Musicians
  relationship with audience, 14–15, 20
Personality, therapeutic, 195
Philosophical Investigations (Wittgenstein), 164, 172
Physical assault, by patient, 192–193
Physics, reality crisis of, 173–174
Popular culture, paranoia of, 94, 96–97
Positivism, logical, 163, 164, 175
Principia Mathematica, The (Russell and Whitehead), 162
Projection
  definition, 226
  by paranoid patients, 90–91, 93
  by terminally ill patients, 127–129, 134
Projective identification, 226–227

Projective testing, of paranoid patients, 95
Psychodrama, 189–190

Quantum mechanics, reality crisis of, 173–174

Radical therapist, 189–191
Rage, narcissistic, 23–24
Raging Bull (film), 96–97
Rationalization, 130–131, 227
Reality, artist's inner world versus, 154–156
Reality crisis, 173–174
Reality testing, 11, 14, 20
Reichman, Frieda Fromm, 185
Religious disciple, 203–204
Remarks on Color (Wittgenstein), 166
Remarks on the Foundations of Mathematics (Wittgenstein), 164
Repression
  definition, 227
  by terminally ill patients, 131
  of trauma, 84–86
Resistance, of patient, 188
Role expectations, 149
Role playing, 153
Role-reversal, in therapist–patient relationship, 48–49, 87–88
Role theory, 203
Roth, Philip, 56
Russell, Bertrand, 162, 163, 166

Sadomasochism, in audience–artist relationship, 19–20
Schizoid defenses, 130, 153
Schizoid personality, 139–156
  artistic inspiration and, 151–152

Schizoid personality (*cont.*)
  case examples, 139–146, 147, 150
  characteristics of, 152–153
  creativity and, 149–150
  defense mechanisms of, 153
  definition, 227
  developmental factors in, 152, 153
  role expectations and, 149
  schizoid thought processes of, 150–151
Schizophrenia, 223
Schlick, Moritz, 161
Schoenburg, Arnold, 161
Schrödinger, Erwin, 174
Scientific hypotheses, falsifiability of, 170
Scorsese, Martin 63
Searles, Harold, 189
Self
  authorial, 185
  false, 10
    of artist, 26
    compliance of, 156
    definition, 224
    falseness of analytic situation and, 185–191
    false therapeutic techniques and, 191–195
    function of, 179–180
    radical therapies and, 189–191
    of therapist, 26, 180–198
    therapist's code of conduct and, 191–194
  grandiose, 12, 14, 15, 224
  second, 185
  suicide of, 7
  supraordinated, 7

Self (*cont.*)
  true, 10
  analyst as, 195–196
  definition, 228
  developmental importance of, 179
Self-analysis, 210
Self-esteem, 11, 218
  externalization of, 13
  internalizational of, 13
  narcissism and, 40
Selfobject
  audience as, 13, 15, 40
  definition, 227–228
  objective, 13, 228
Self psychology, 40
Sexual relations, with patient, 191
Shapiro, David, 226
Smythies, Yorick, 166
Splitting of the ego, 9–10, 129–130, 228
Strategic therapy, 211–212
Success, of the artist, 217–220
Suicide
  as denial of death, 134
  fantasies of, 79–81
Symbiosis
  death as, 130
  definition, 228

Talent, artistic
  artist's attitude toward, 7–10
  artist's relationship to, 7–15
  during therapy, 7–12
  as grandiose self, 12
  transference and, 7–9, 11–12
  transformative nature of, 6–7
Taxi Driver (film), 96–97

Temperament, artistic, schizoid personality and, 139, 146, 149–156
Terminally ill patient, 101–135
  countertransference with, 109
  death of, 121–122
  defense mechanisms of, 122–135
    adaptive defenses, 125, 126
    ego splitting, 129–130
    intellectualization, 126–127
    paranoid defenses, 129
    projection, 127–129
    rationalization, 130–131
    repression, 131
    schizoid defenses, 130
  denial of death by, 113, 117, 118, 122–124, 127, 133, 222
  depression of, 101–103, 108, 111, 113
  empathy of, 124
  existential philosophy of, 127
  illness of, 111–121
  life history of, 103–108, 109–111
  projection by, 134
  psychological well-being of, 120, 125
  termination of therapy by, 121, 122
Termination, of therapy, 37–39, 121, 122
Theatricality, of artist's interpersonal relationships, 40, 154–156
Therapist
  artistic tastes of, 9, 11–12
  attitude toward artist-patients, 9, 11–12
  code of conduct, 191–194

Therapist (cont.)
  eclectic, 190–191
  false self, 180–198
    code of conduct and, 191–194
    examples of, 180–183
    falseness of analytic situation and, 185–191
    false techniques and, 191–195
    of radical therapists, 189–191
    "good enough," 197–198
  patient's attitude toward, 7–9
  radical, 189–191
  second self, 185
  true self, 195
Therapist–patient relationship. See also Countertransference; Transference; Double bind, therapeutic
  aggression in, 191–193
  code of conduct regarding, 191–194
  patient's artistic talent and, 7–9
  sexual relations in, 191
Therapy training institutes
  candidates' training in, 196
  false self analysts and, 180–184
Thinking
  grandiose, 78–79
  paranoid, 84–86, 94, 95
  schizoid, 150–151
Tough Guys (film), 23–24
Tractatus Logico-Philosophicus, The (Wittgenstein), 162–164, 168, 169, 172, 174, 175
Transference, 7–8
  double bind and, 212–213
  effects of, 212–213
  interpersonal fragmentation and, 187

Transference (cont.)
  intimacy and, 213
  narcissism and, 8
  negative, 8, 12, 188
  as normal therapeutic response, 187
  with paranoid patient, 86, 97
  patient's artistic talent and, 7–9, 11–12
  positive, 8, 11–12
  selfobject and, 39–40
Trauma
  effect on drug addiction, 64, 66–68
  of language, 165–166
  repressed, as paranoia, 84–86
Trilling, Lionel, 159
Truth tables, of Wittgenstein, 163

Uncertainty, obsessional, 225–226
Unconscious, of the artist, 150–151, 152
Unemployment, of artists, 148

Vinci, Leonardo da, 160
Violence
  popular cultural depictions of, 96
  during therapy sessions, 191–194

Waiters, artists' employment as, 22–24, 148
Whitehead, Alfred North, 162, 163
Winnicott, D. W., 179–180, 183, 185, 191, 197, 198, 224, 228
Wittgenstein, Ludwig, 159–176
  The Blue and Brown Books, 164
  Freud and, 171–173
  language theory of, 163, 164, 165–166, 168–176
  psychoanalysis and, 169–176
  logical atomism of, 164, 168
  logical positivism and, 163, 164, 175
  paranoid style of, 161, 166–169
  Philosophical Investigations, 164, 172
  prose style of, 159–160, 171–173
  Remarks on Color, 166
  Remarks on the Foundations of Mathematics, 164
  The Tractatus Logico-Philosophicus, 162–164, 168, 169, 172, 174, 175
  truth tables of, 163
Work inhibition, 7, 148, 152